Scan the QR code
to read and listen to the
glossary words for FREE!

glossary - Meanings of words.

Published in the UK by Every Cherry Publishing Limited, 2025
Unit 36, Vulcan House, Vulcan Road,
Leicester LE5 3EF, United Kingdom

Unit 31, The Pottery, Bakers Point,
Pottery Road, Dún Laoghaire,
Dublin A96 EV18, Ireland

2 4 6 8 10 9 7 5 3 1

ISBN: 978-1-80263-673-4

Easier Classics
King Lear

Based on the original play by William Shakespeare.
Adapted by Gemma Barder and Christian Emmerson.
Illustrations by Mai Ngo.

www.everycherry.com

Printed and bound in China

MIX
Paper | Supporting responsible forestry
FSC® C188448
FSC www.fsc.org

Every Cherry

King Lear

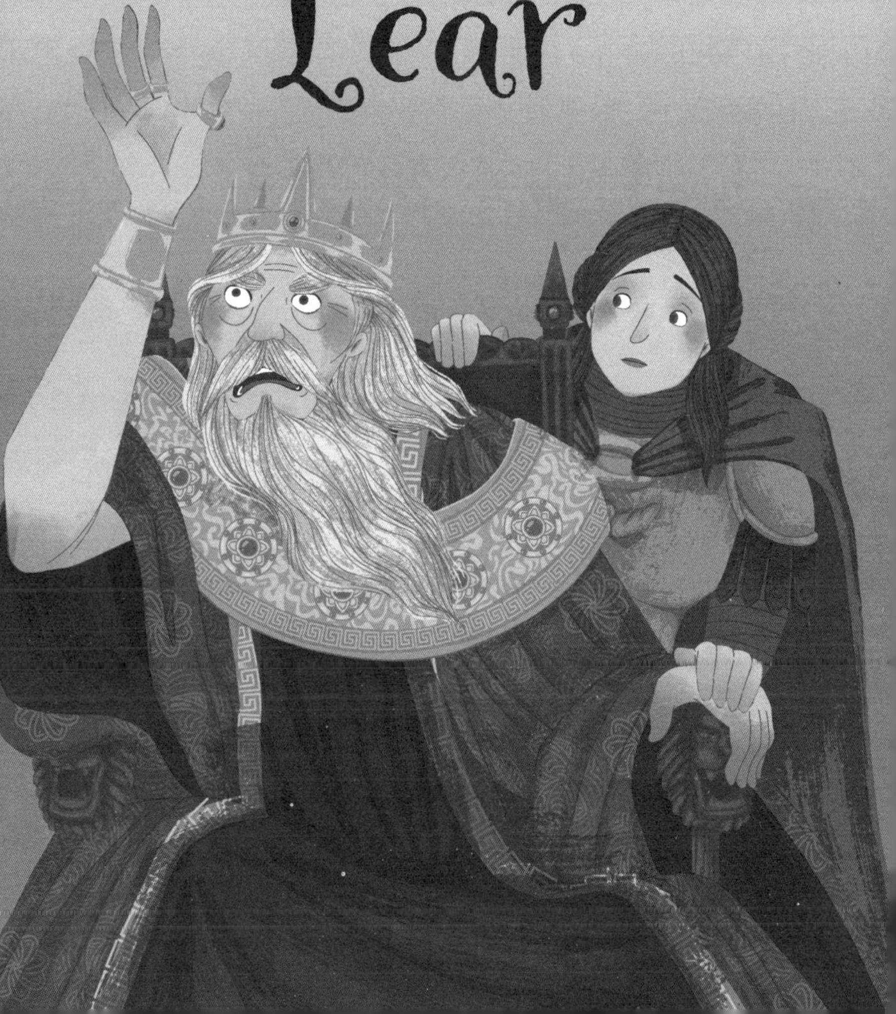

Meet the Characters

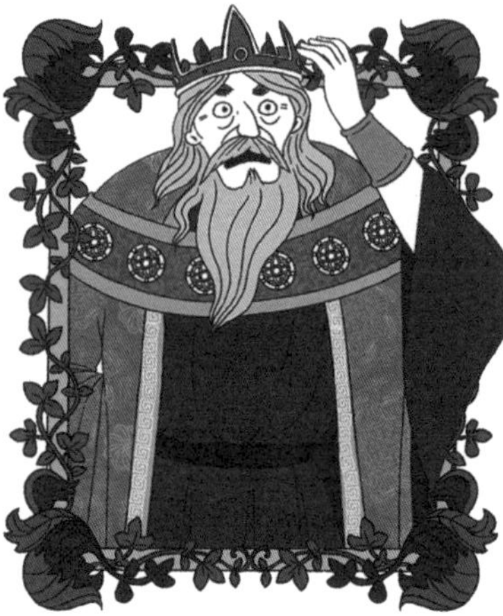

King Lear

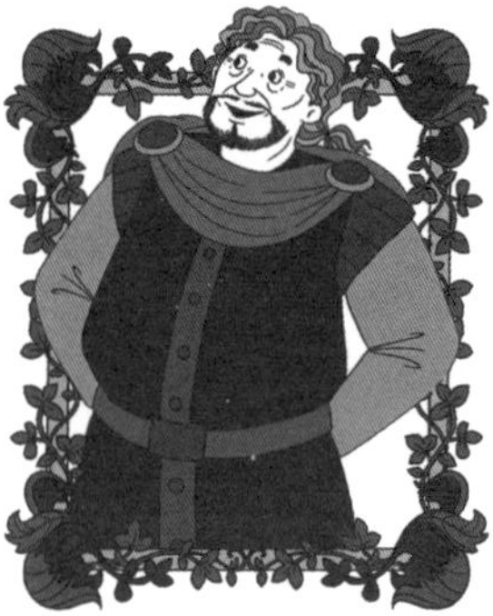

Kent

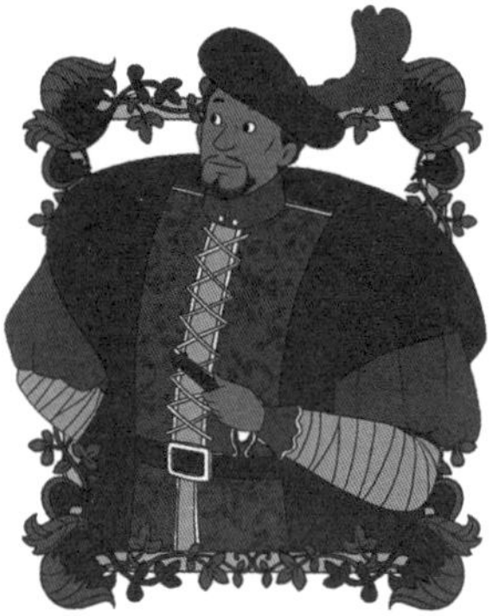

King of France

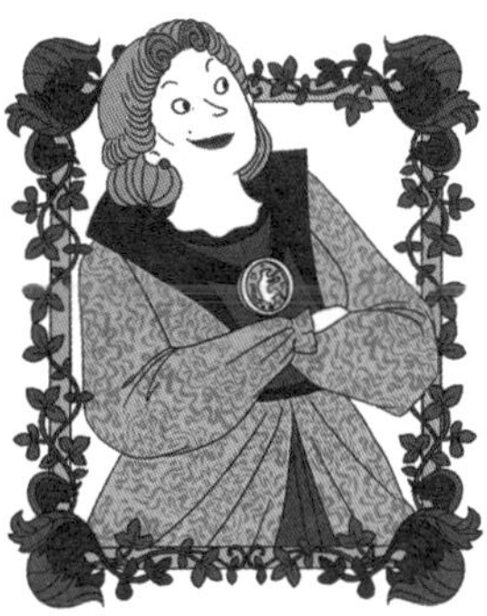

Goneril

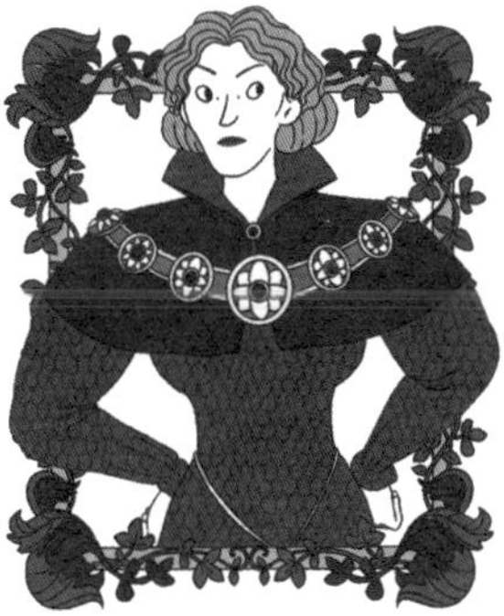

Regan

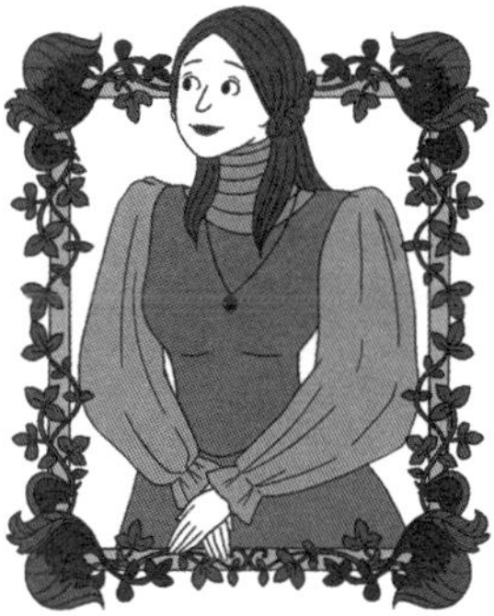

Cordelia

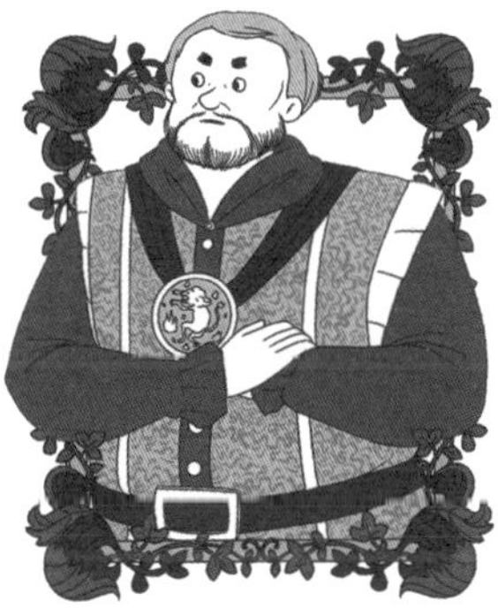

Albany

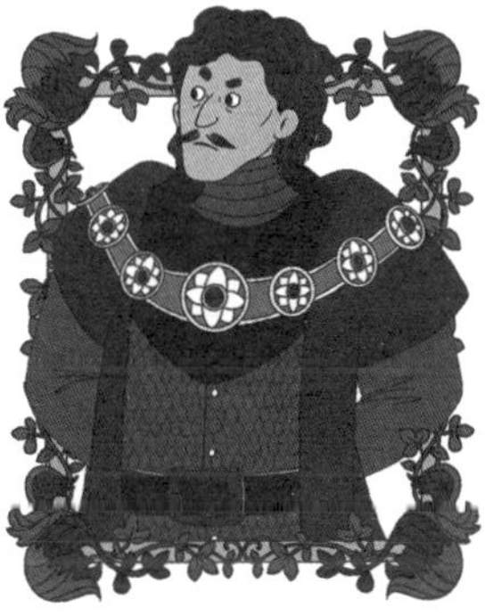

Cornwall

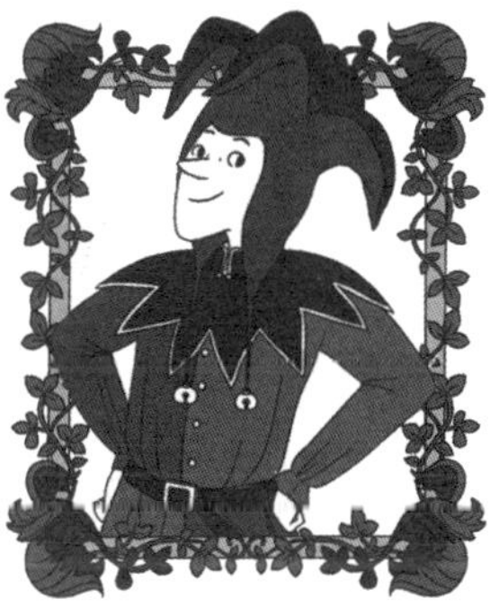

Jester

Chapter 1

King Lear was sitting on his throne. His old friend, the **Duke** of Kent, and his **jester** were with him.

King Lear was a good king, but he was an old man now.

'What happened to the brave young man I used to be?' King Lear asked.

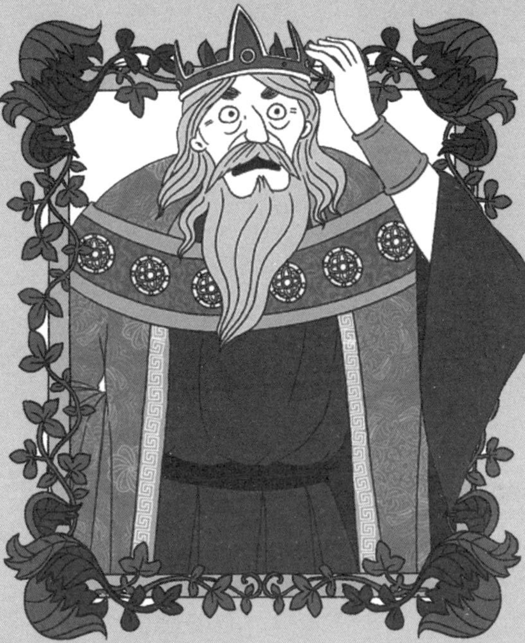

Duke - An important man with power in an area of the country, usually working closely with the royal family.

jester - Someone whose job was to do silly things to make people laugh, a bit like a clown.

'You became a wise and much-loved king,' said Kent.

'What do you think, jester?' asked King Lear. 'Am I wise and loved?'

The jester danced over to the King. 'Let me check, Your **Majesty**!'

He skipped around King Lear, poking him and looking into his ears.

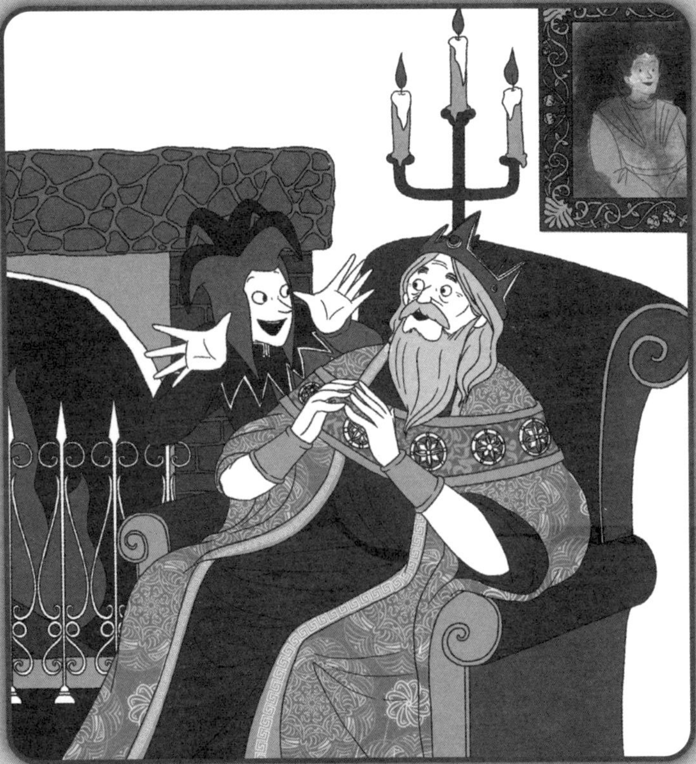

Majesty - A word you can call a king or queen when talking to or about them.

King Lear laughed and shooed the jester away.

'I have an idea,' King Lear said.

Kent stepped closer.

'I want to stop being king.
My **kingdom** of England will go to my three daughters,' King Lear said. 'I will split the **kingdom** between them.'

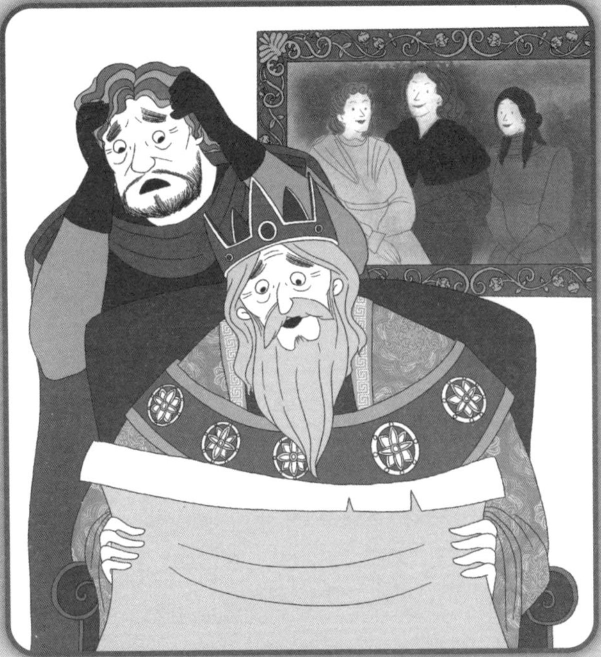

kingdom - *A place that is ruled by a king or queen.*

'Are you sure, Your Majesty?' Kent asked. 'Some parts of the kingdom are better than others. How will you choose which daughter gets the best part?'

'Simple!' King Lear said. 'I shall ask each of them how much they love me.'

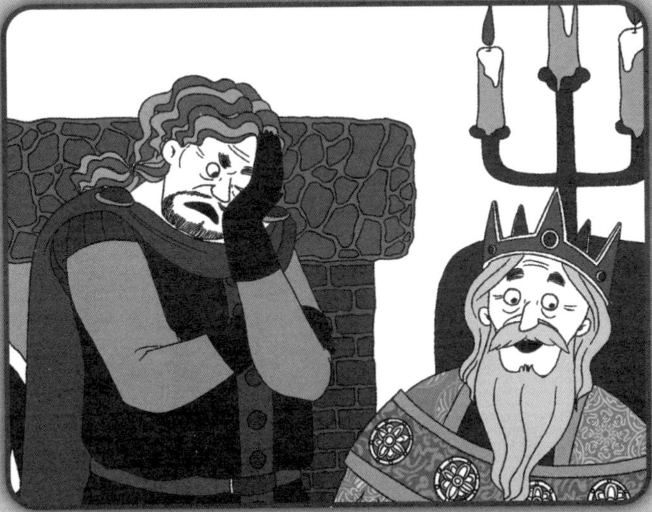

'The best part of the kingdom will go to the daughter who loves me the most,' King Lear said.

Kent thought King Lear's plan seemed silly. He thought the kingdom should be ruled by the daughter who was the best leader.

Kent was worried about King Lear. He did not seem himself.

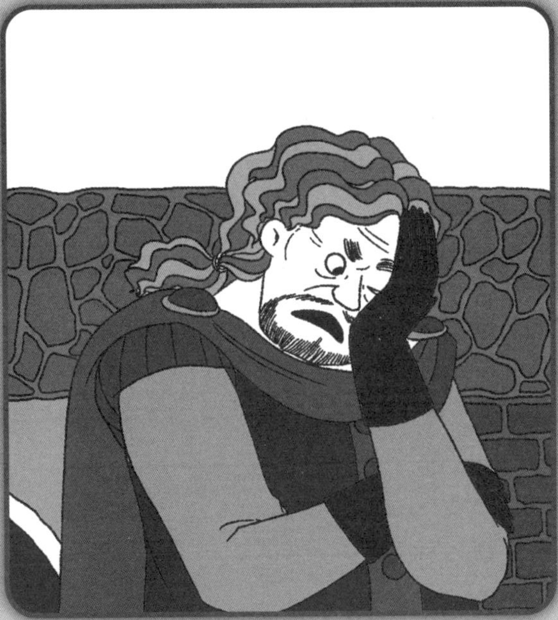

'Your Majesty, are you sure?' Kent asked. 'Maybe you should think about it more.'

Kent thought King Lear was making a bad choice.

'No!' King Lear shouted. 'The time for thinking is over. Get my daughters at once.'

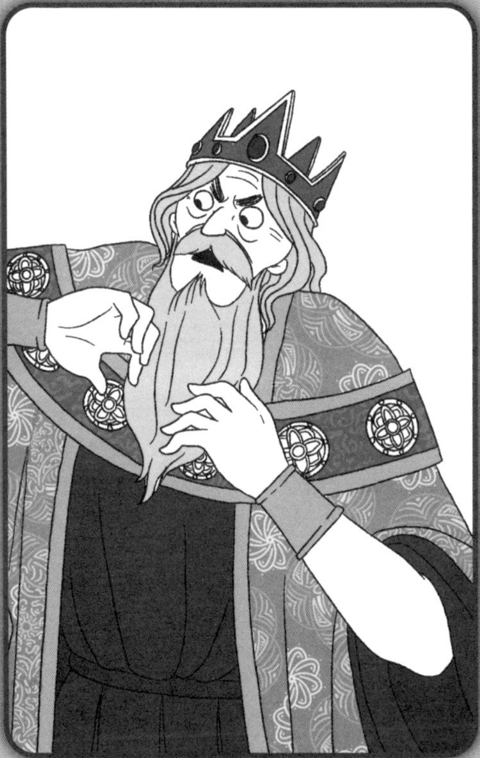

Chapter 2

Kent sent out two **messengers**.

One went to King Lear's eldest daughter, Goneril, and her husband, the Duke of Albany.

The other went to his middle daughter, Regan, and her husband, the Duke of Cornwall.

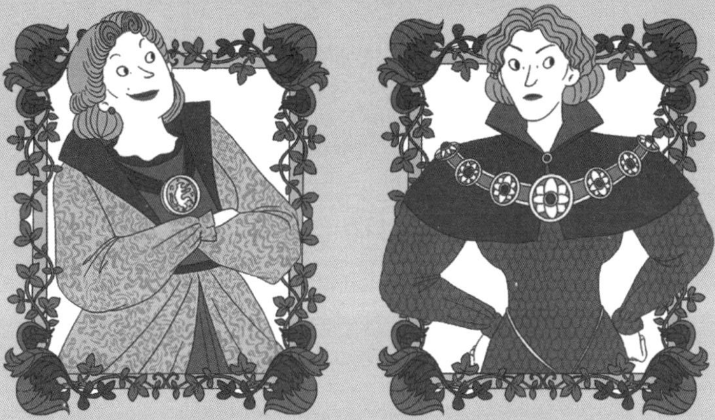

messengers - People who take messages to someone as their job.

King Lear's youngest daughter, Cordelia, still lived with him.

The King of France had fallen in love with Cordelia. He had asked her to marry him, and she had said yes.

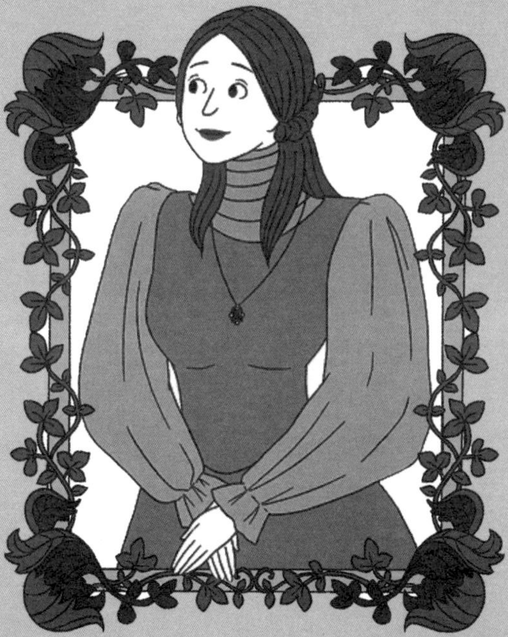

King Lear had decided to tell the people in his kingdom the news. Many people had come to hear King Lear talk.

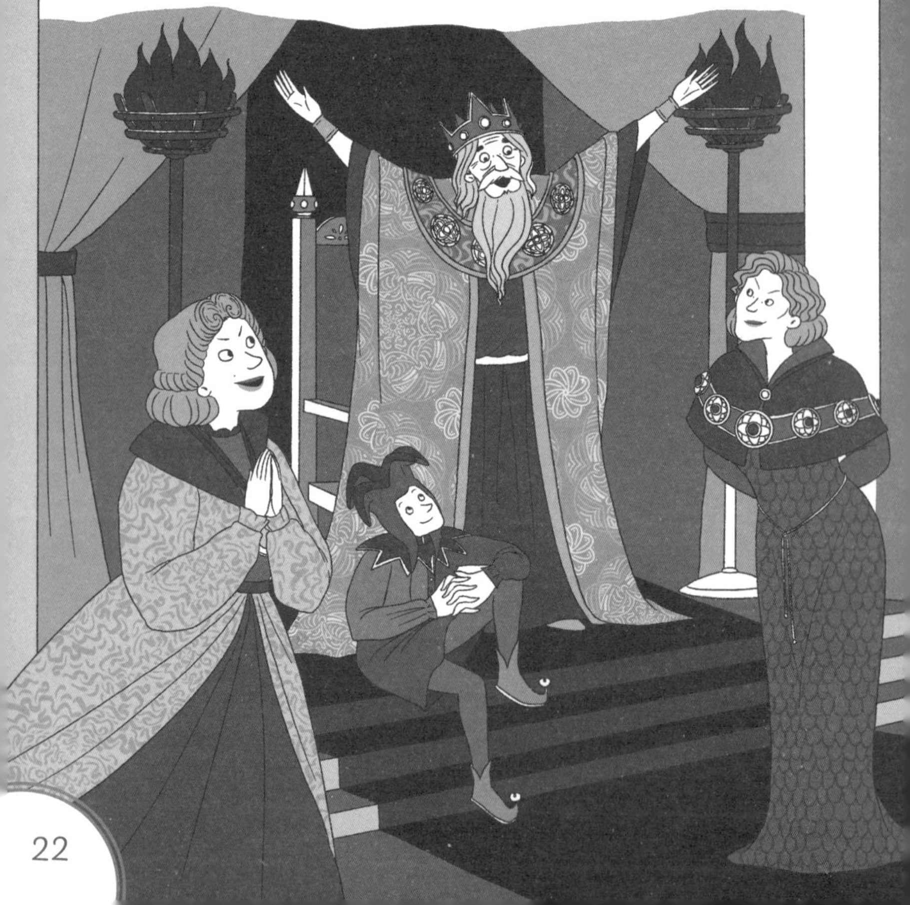

'Welcome everyone,' King Lear said. 'I have enjoyed ruling this great kingdom for many years. I am old and tired. It is time for someone younger to rule.'

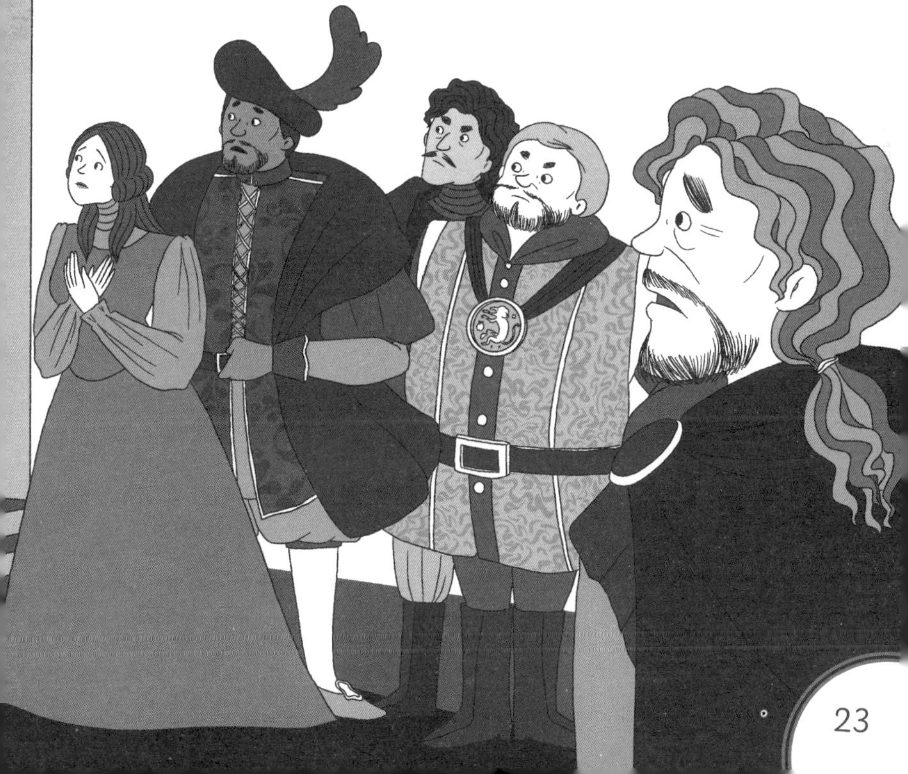

'I have decided to split the kingdom into three parts,' said King Lear. 'Each part is to be ruled by one of my daughters.'

Goneril and Regan looked very happy.

But Cordelia was confused. She looked at her father's friend, Kent. He looked worried and shook his head.

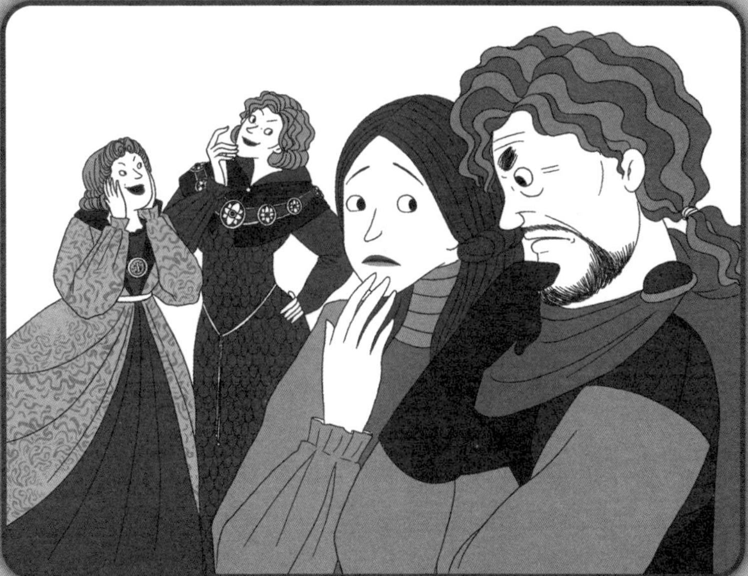

'To decide which part of the kingdom goes to which daughter, I will ask you a simple question,' said King Lear. 'How much do you love me?'

Goneril stepped forward first. She kneeled at King Lear's feet.

'Dear Father,' she said. 'I love you more than words can say. I love you more than life itself!'

King Lear smiled at his eldest daughter.

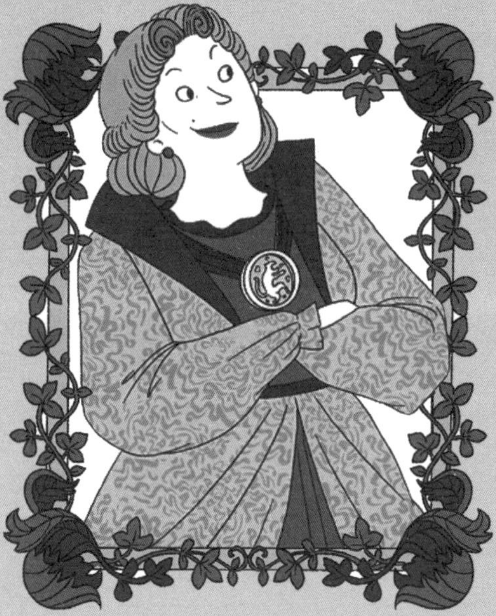

Next, Regan stepped forward. She hugged King Lear and began to cry.

'Oh Father!' she said. 'My love for you is brighter than the sun.'

King Lear looked very happy indeed.

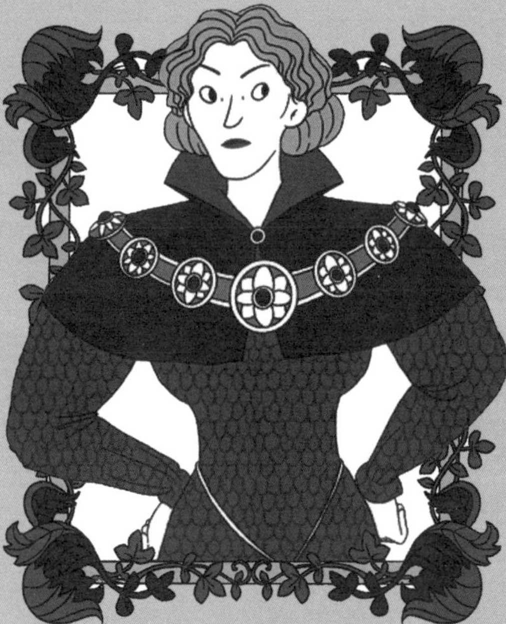

'I can't speak in front of all of these people!' whispered Cordelia to the King of France.

'Don't you love your father?' questioned the King of France.

'Of course I do,' Cordelia said. 'Very much.'

'Then you must try,' said the King of France.

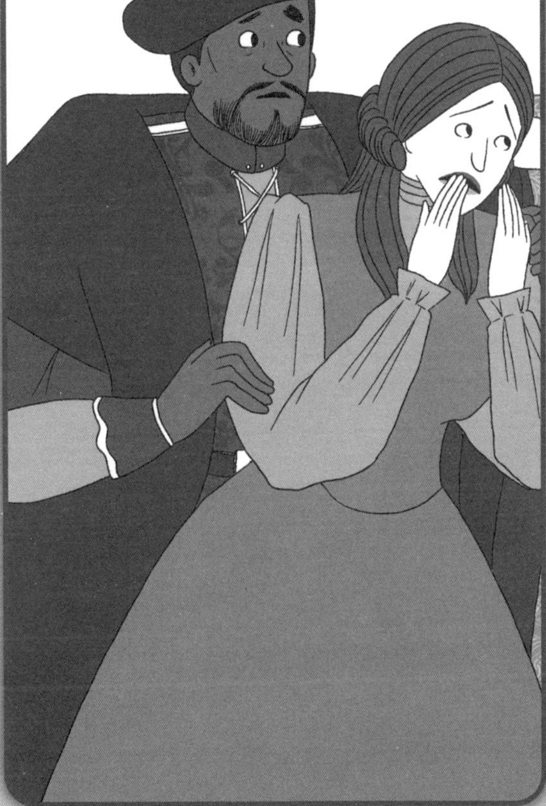

Chapter 3

Cordelia was nervous. She knelt before her father. She looked into his eyes but couldn't speak.

'How will I know how much you love me if you don't speak?' said King Lear.

'All I can say is that my love for you is true and real,' Cordelia said.

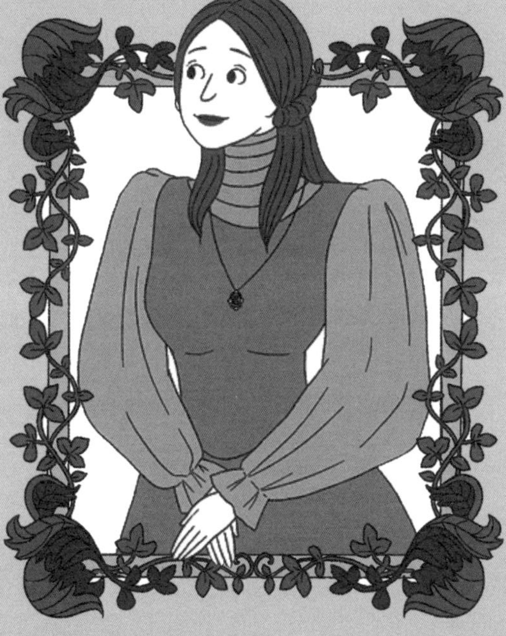

King Lear stared at Cordelia.

He looked confused and upset.

'Is that all you have to say?' he said.

Cordelia nodded.

King Lear's face turned red with anger.

'Then Goneril and Regan will rule over half of the kingdom each!' he shouted.

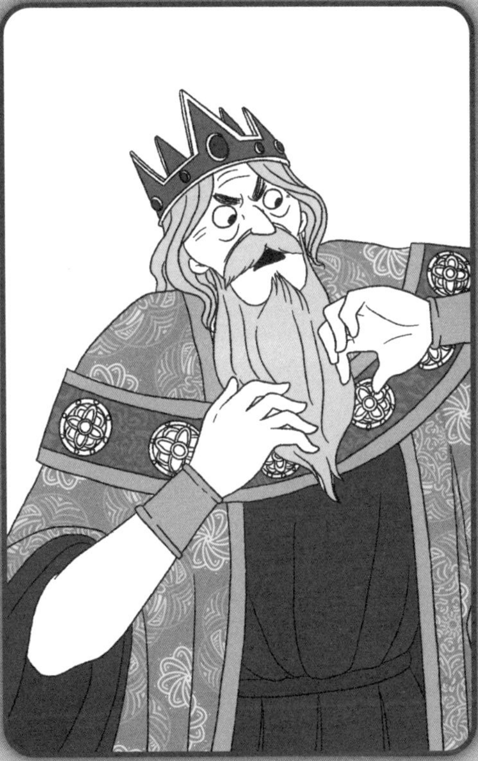

King Lear looked at Cordelia.

'You are not my daughter anymore.

Leave and never come back!' he said.

Cordelia was heartbroken.

'Your Majesty, Cordelia loves you,'

said Kent. 'She is just shy.'

'If you believe that, you do not love

me either!' King Lear said.

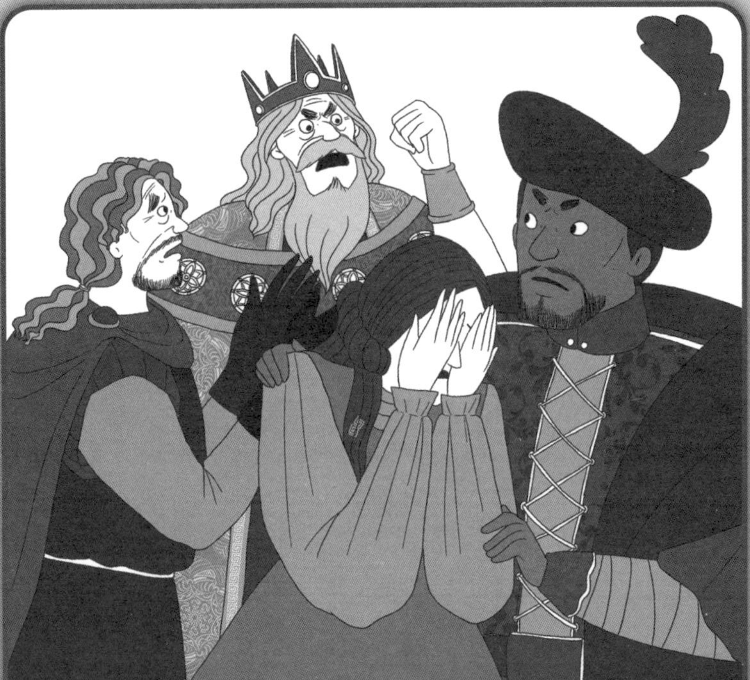

King Lear turned to the King of France.

'My daughter is an **ungrateful** woman,' he said. 'You should stop the wedding.'

The King of France was shocked at King Lear's comment.

'I love Cordelia more than ever,' the King of France said. 'She may not be welcome here, but she is welcome in France.'

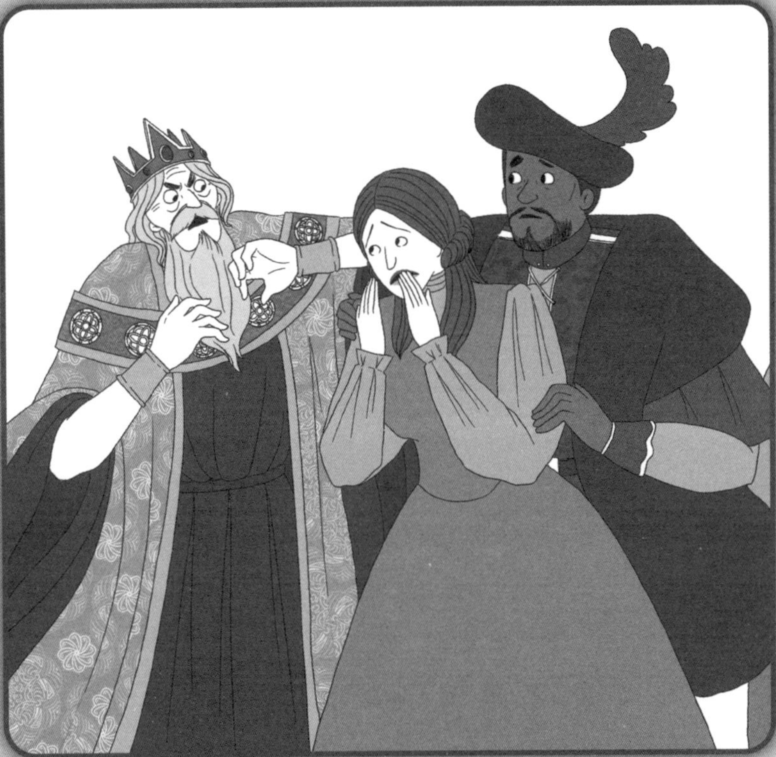

ungrateful - To not show thanks for something or to someone.

Cordelia stood still, staring at her father in shock. The room had fallen silent.

Her sisters were smiling **greedily**. They couldn't wait to take over the kingdom.

The King of France took Cordelia's hand. They left the room. They decided to leave the castle and move to France straight away.

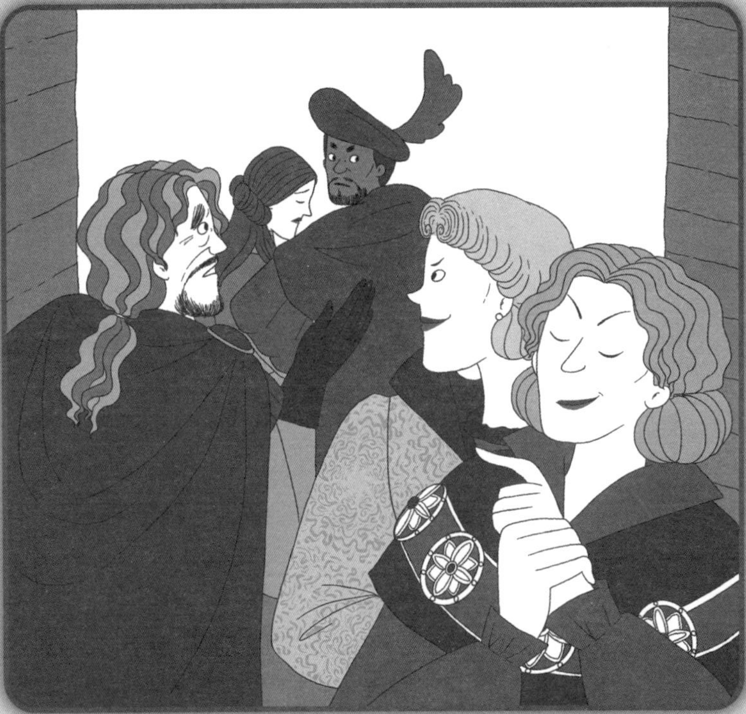

greedily - Wanting too much of something, like food or money.

Kent watched Cordelia go.

'Your Majesty,' he said to King Lear, 'please don't do this.'

'Don't tell me what to do, Kent!' King Lear shouted. 'You are **banished** from the kingdom. I never want to see you again!'

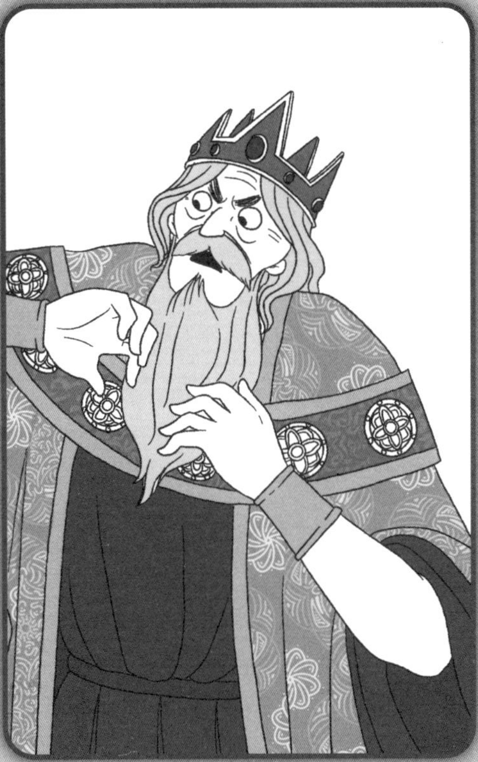

banished - When someone is made to leave a place and not allowed back.

Chapter 4

'You are now in charge of the kingdom,' Lear said to his daughters, Goneril and Regan. 'All I want is 100 **knights** to protect me, a servant, and a **loyal** jester.'

'Of course, Father!' said Goneril, smiling.

'What a good idea,' said Regan.

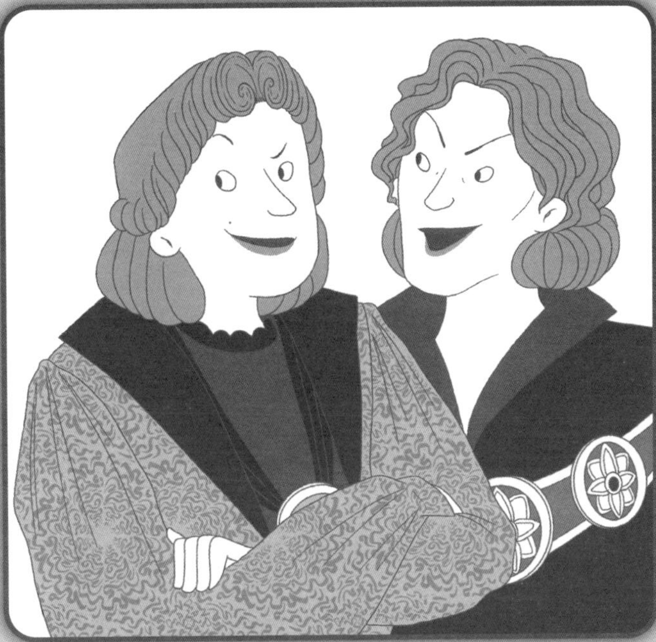

knights - Hundreds of years ago, soldiers who protected or fought for their king or queen.

loyal - Someone who is always a good friend or always shows support for a person or thing.

King Lear did not see that his greedy daughters only cared about money and power.

'Now that I am **retired**,' he said, 'I will live half of the time with you, Goneril, and the other half with you, Regan.'

Goneril and Regan were no longer smiling. They did not want King Lear to live with them at all.

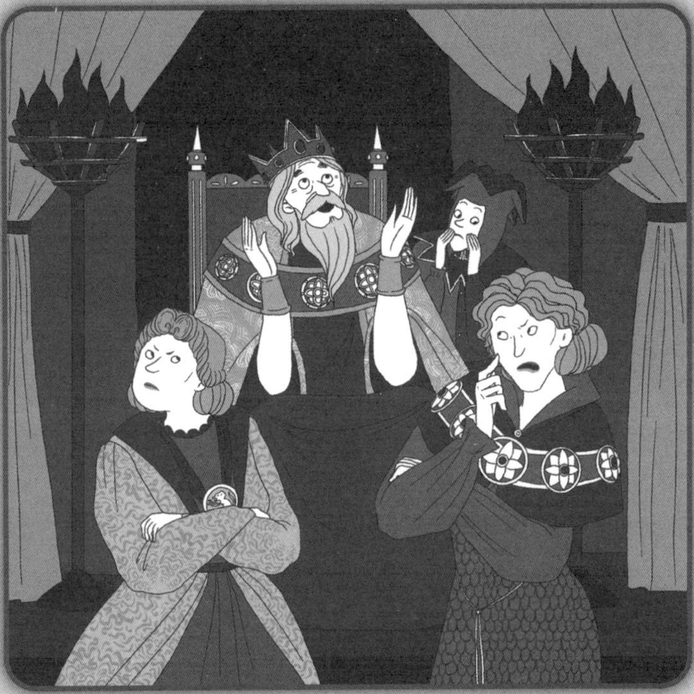

retired - An older person who has left their job and has stopped working completely.

That night, when the guests had left, Goneril went to see Regan.

She knocked on her bedroom door and walked in. Regan looked angry.

'Our father, the old **fool**, wants to live with us,' Goneril said. 'He will always be telling us what to do!'

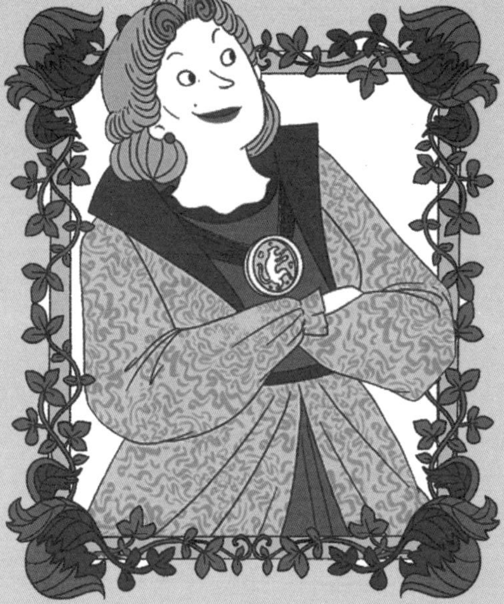

fool - *Someone who is not sensible and who makes silly choices.*

'Then we must stop our father living with us as soon as we can!' Regan said.

'How?' asked Goneril.

'We both know he loved Cordelia more than us,' Regan said. 'But he banished her! He is not thinking clearly. Surely we can **out-think** an old man.'

Goneril smiled. 'I think you might be right,' she said.

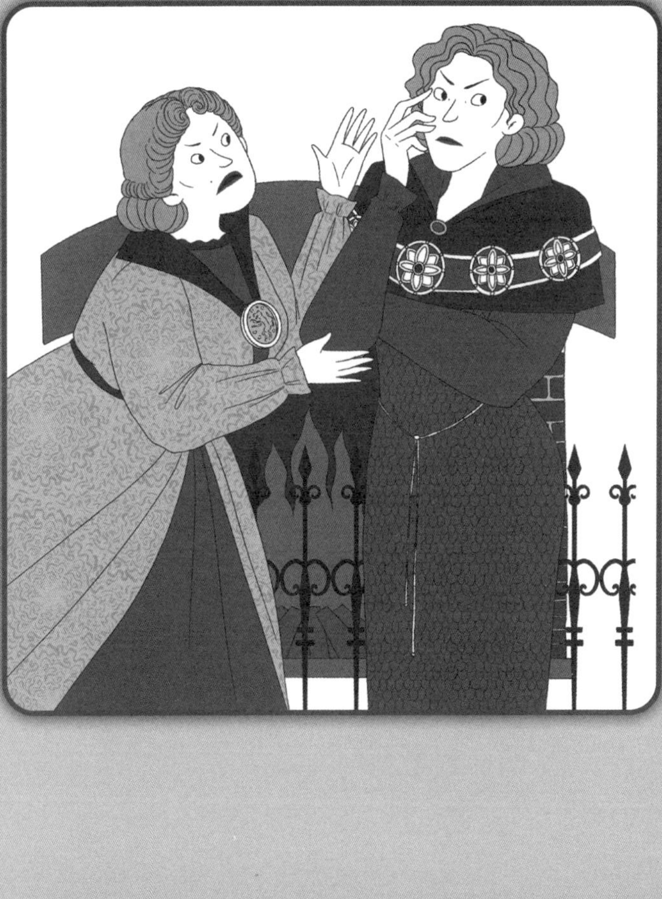

out-think - *To think in a more clever way than someone else.*

Chapter 5

Cordelia was walking in the gardens of her palace in **Paris**. It had been months since her father had banished her.

She was now married to the King of France. But she could not stop thinking about her father.

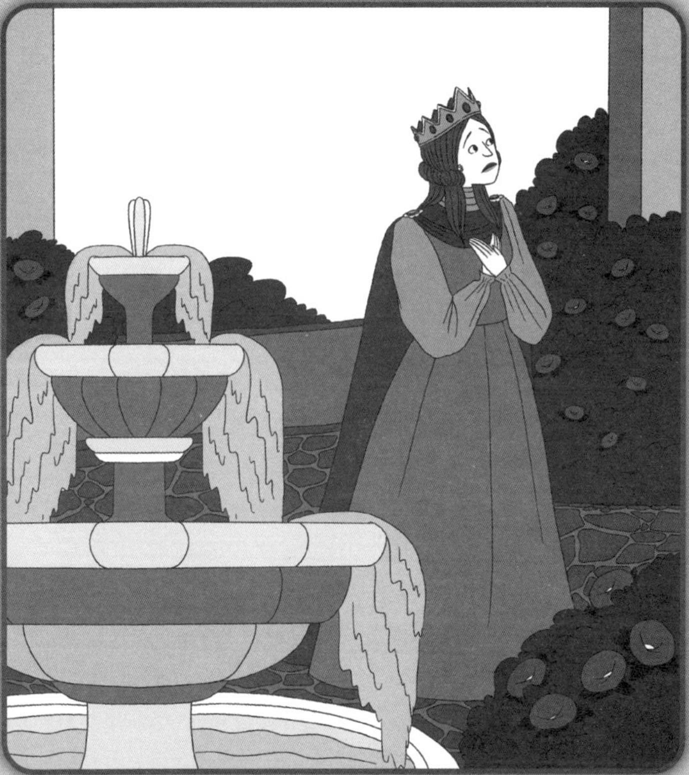

Paris - The capital city of France.

'Your Majesty!' called a familiar voice. It was Kent.

He had been banished for defending Cordelia. So, she had offered him a home with her at her palace in Paris.

'I am sorry for interrupting your walk,' said Kent. 'I have news from home.'

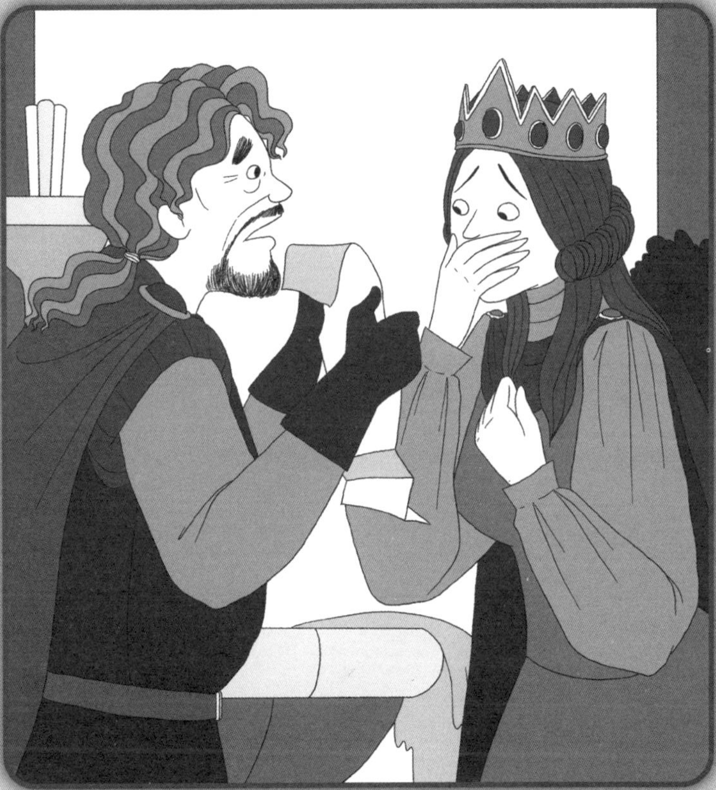

'My friends say your sisters are not good rulers. They are selfish and greedy and do not care about the people at all,' Kent said.

Cordelia sighed.

'My sisters only care about themselves,' she said.

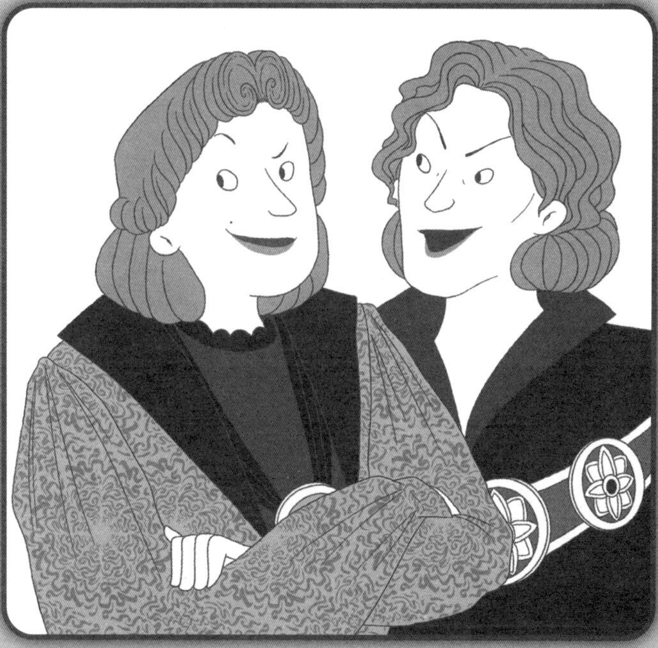

'Your sisters have grown tired of your father,' said Kent. 'He takes it in turn to live with each of them. They don't listen to his **advice**. People say they plan to get rid of him forever.'

Cordelia loved her father very much. She did not want any harm to come to him.

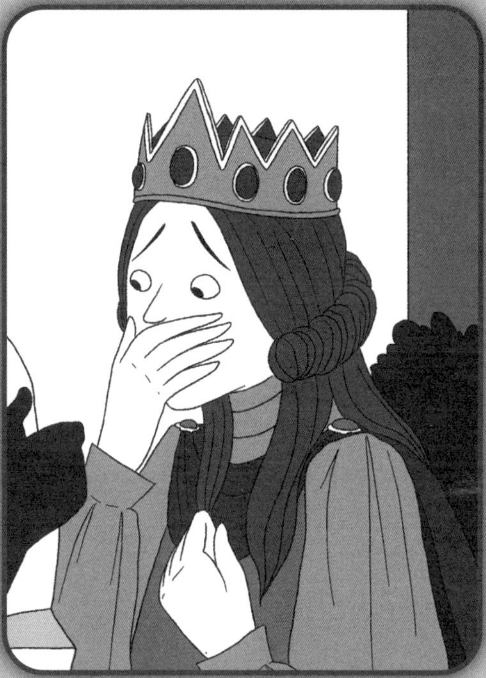

advice *- Ideas on what would be best for someone to do.*

'I am going back to England,' said Kent. 'I will **disguise** myself as a servant and try to get close to your father.'

'My husband and I will follow with an army,' Cordelia said. 'If we cannot save the kingdom from my sisters, then at least we can save my father.'

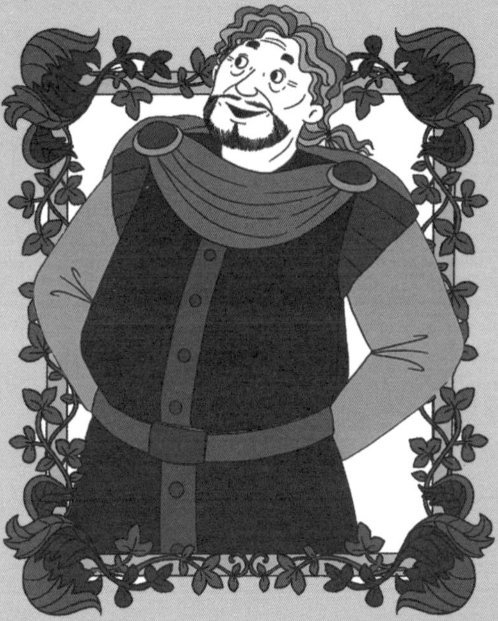

disguise - Change how you look so that you can't be recognised.

Kent travelled back to England before Cordelia.

He was disguised so well that he tricked everyone around him!

He began working as King Lear's new servant.

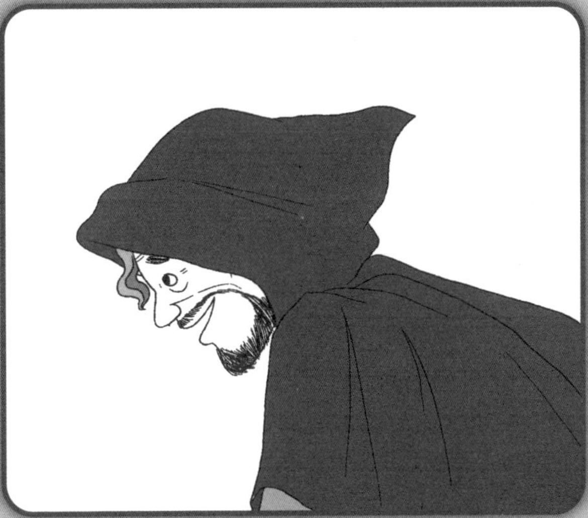

One day, Kent, disguised as King Lear's new servant, was helping the king.

'Thank you,' King Lear said. 'You have only been with me for a few days but you are one of the best servants I have ever had!' said King Lear.

Kent smiled. His disguise had worked.

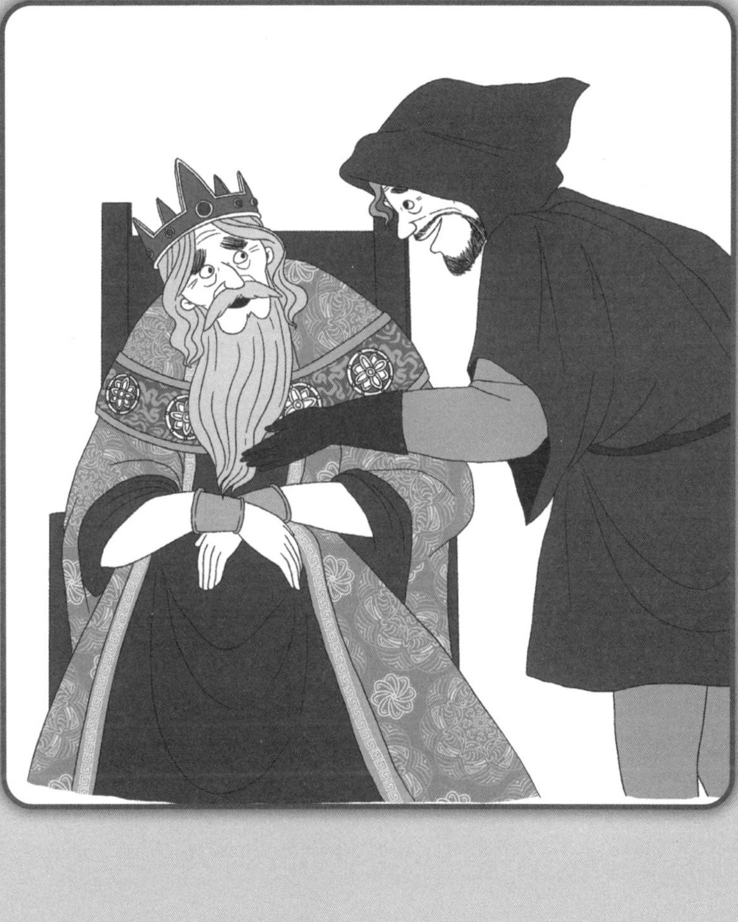

Chapter 6

Goneril **slammed** her bedroom door behind her. 'I can't take it anymore!' she screamed at her husband.

'What is wrong?' he asked.

'My father! The stables are full of his knights' horses,' she said. 'The castle is full of his knights. He is always telling me what to do!'

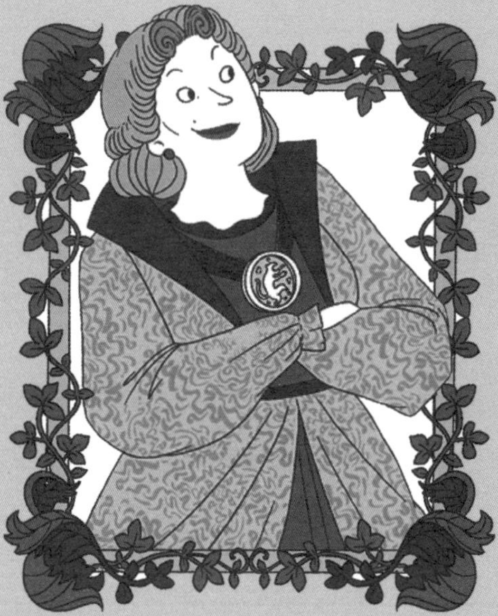

slammed - Shut something very loudly.

At that moment, there was a knock on the bedroom door. Without waiting for a reply, King Lear walked in.

'There you are, Goneril,' he said. 'I have to talk to you about these new **taxes** you are making our people pay. People have no money!'

Goneril sighed.

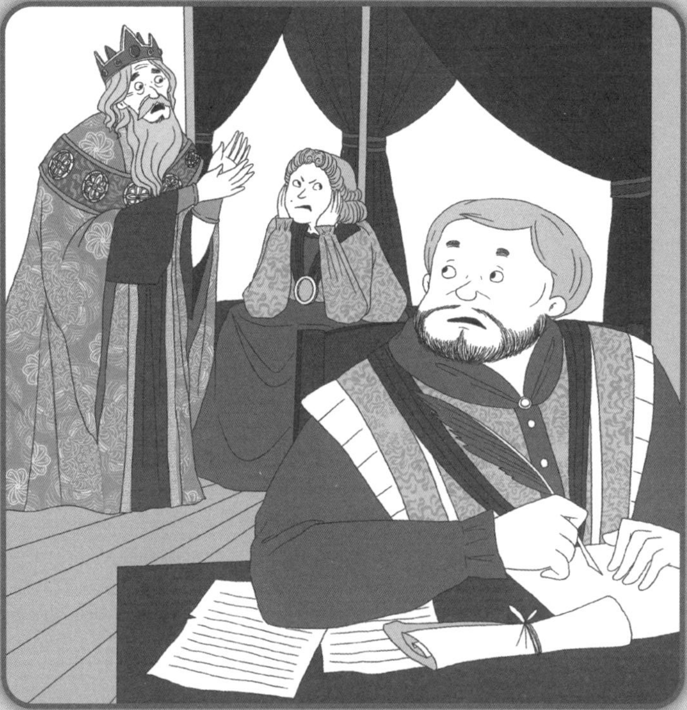

taxes - *Money paid to the government to pay for things like roads, schools, and hospitals. Hundreds of years ago, this money would have been paid to the king or queen.*

King Lear carried on talking.

'My knights say your stable boys aren't giving my horses much to eat!' King Lear said.

Goneril smiled.

'Well, Father, there is a reason for that,' she said. 'You have so many people with you, it's hard to feed everyone. I had to raise the taxes to pay for your visits.'

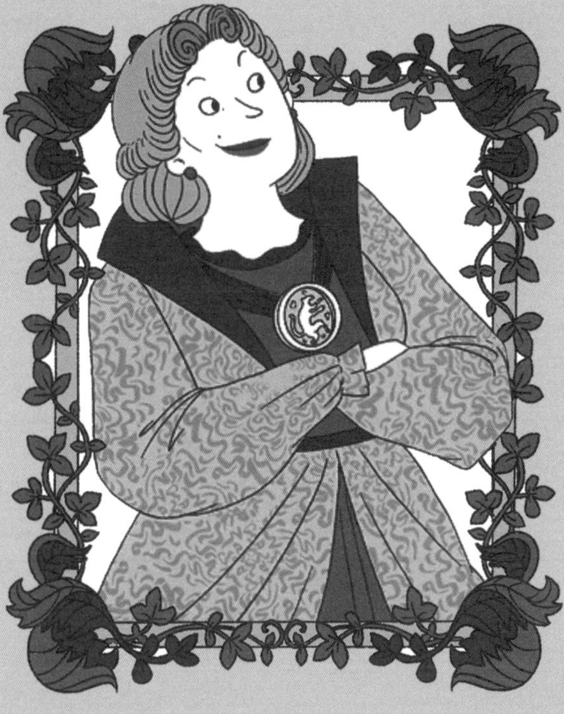

Of course, none of this was true.

Goneril had raised taxes because she wanted more money. She had plenty of food to feed everyone.

'Oh dear,' said King Lear, looking confused. 'What should we do?'

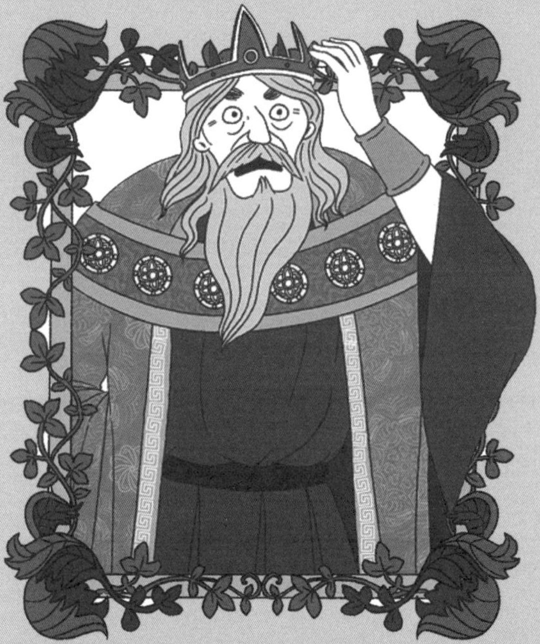

'Perhaps you could have fifty knights instead of 100,' Goneril said.

King Lear nodded. 'Well, if you really think I should ...' he said.

'I do!' said Goneril. 'Why don't you go and tell them now, before you go to visit Regan?'

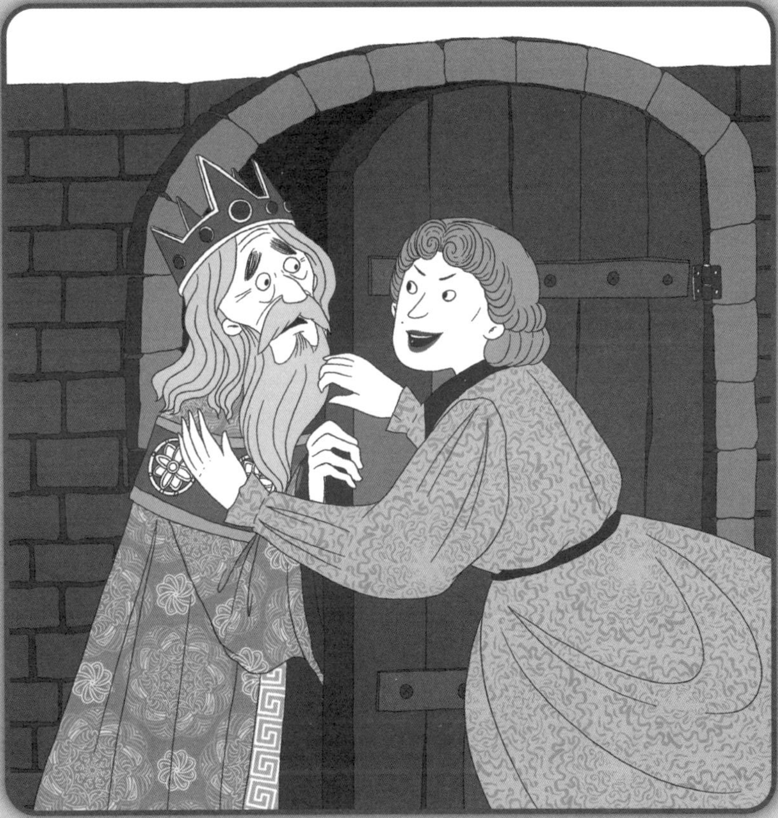

Goneril shut the door.

'That was easy,' she said. 'The old fool will do anything I say!'

'Very clever,' Albany said. 'But he still has fifty knights ready to defend him.'

'Not for long!' Goneril said. She sat at her table and wrote a letter to her sister.

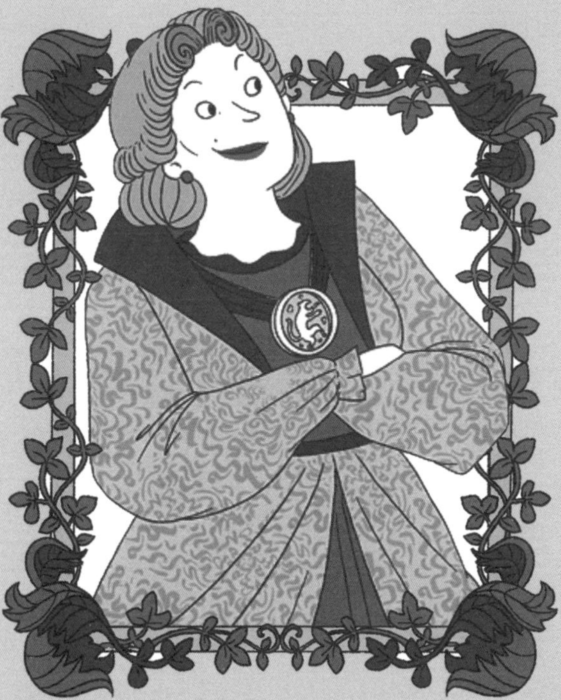

Chapter 7

Regan read the letter from Goneril.

'Goneril has a plan!' she said to her husband.

'For what?' asked Cornwall, looking up from his breakfast.

'To get rid of my father!'

Regan handed the letter to her husband to read.

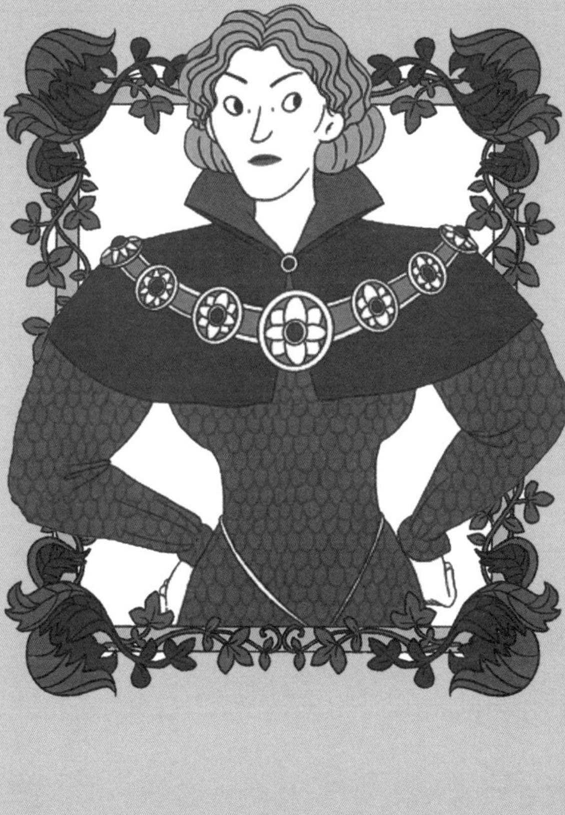

Dearest sister,

I have told Father to get rid of half his knights. You must tell him the same.

Tell him you can't afford to feed them. He must get rid of everyone.

Then all that will stand in our way is his silly old jester and his new servant!

From Goneril

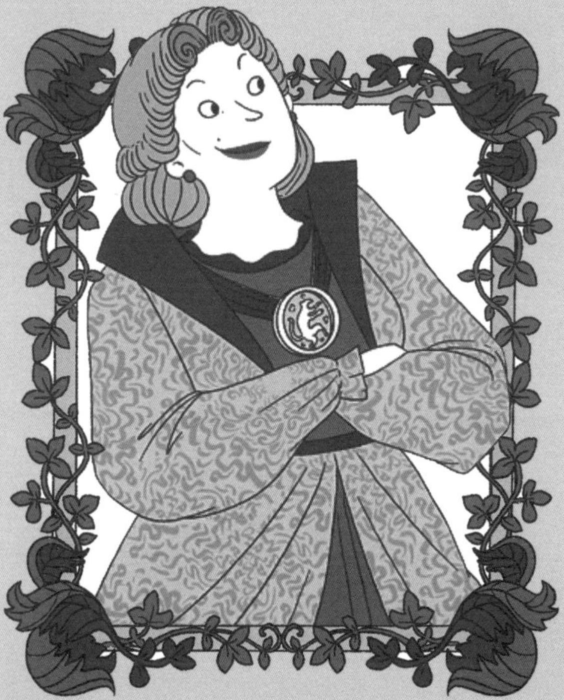

'Isn't it a great plan?' Regan asked, as Cornwall finished reading the letter.

'My dear, your sister is **obsessed** with getting rid of your father,' he said.

'He gets in the way,' Regan said crossly. 'Goneril wants to be in control, just like I do.'

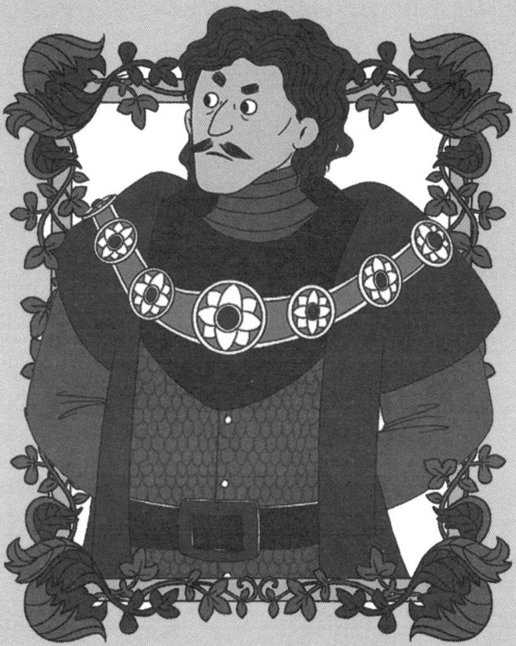

obsessed - Constantly thinking about one thing and finding it difficult to think about anything else.

'But what will she do when King Lear is gone?' asked Cornwall.

Regan frowned. 'What do you mean?' she asked.

'What if your sister wants to take over all of the kingdom for herself?' asked Cornwall.

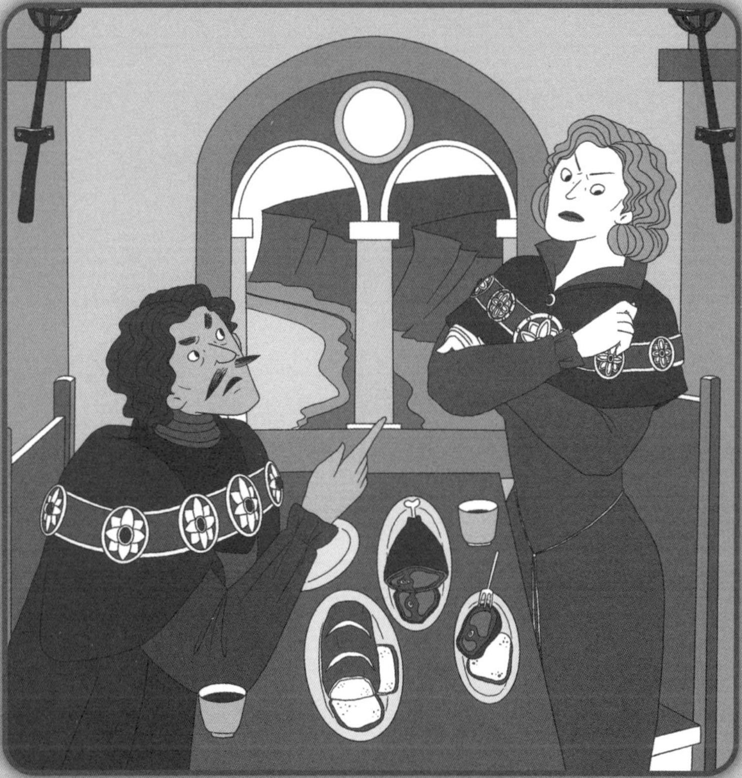

Later, King Lear watched the last of his knights leave.

'Your Majesty,' said Kent quietly. 'Is everything all right?'

'My trusted knights have all gone,' King Lear said sadly.

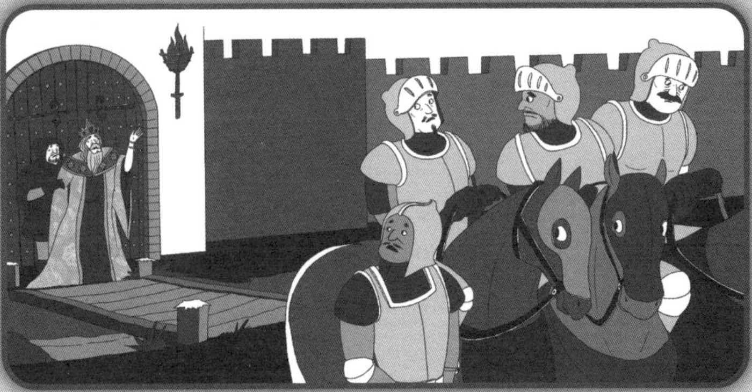

Kent knew exactly what Goneril and Regan were up to. He knew they were trying to get rid of King Lear so they could rule the kingdom without him.

Kent had known them since they were little girls. They had grown up to be **selfish**, greedy women.

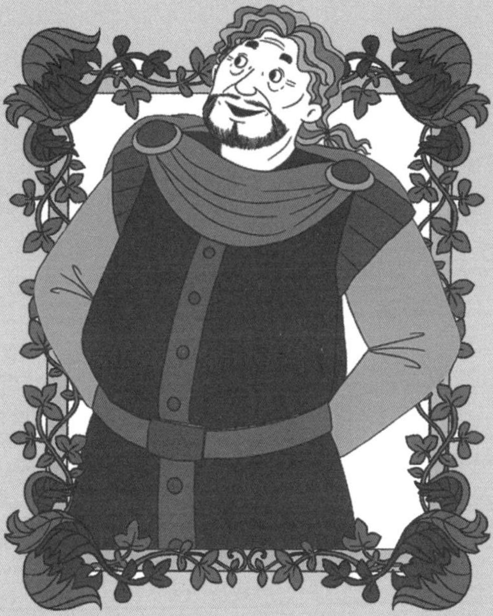

selfish - *Only caring about themselves.*

'What will you do now, King Lear?' asked Kent.

King Lear looked up towards the castle.

'I will go back inside and see my daughter,' King Lear said. 'At least I still have two loyal daughters left.'

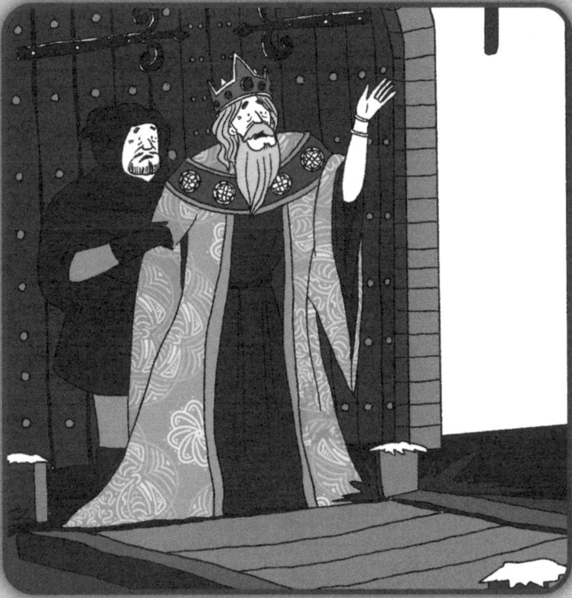

King Lear turned to the huge entrance of Regan's castle.

There were no guards to let him in.

He banged his fist on the door, but there was no reply.

King Lear was locked out of the castle.

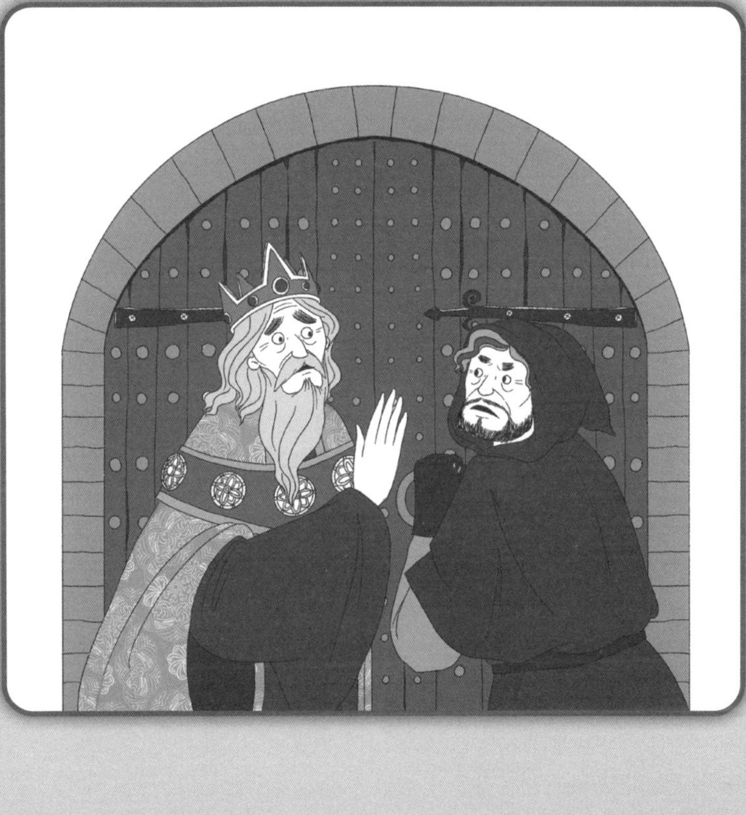

Chapter 8

King Lear, the jester and Kent, still disguised as a servant, walked along a dark road.

'Night-time is coming, but there are no knights to be seen!' the jester sang. 'Poor old King Lear is left out in the cold!'

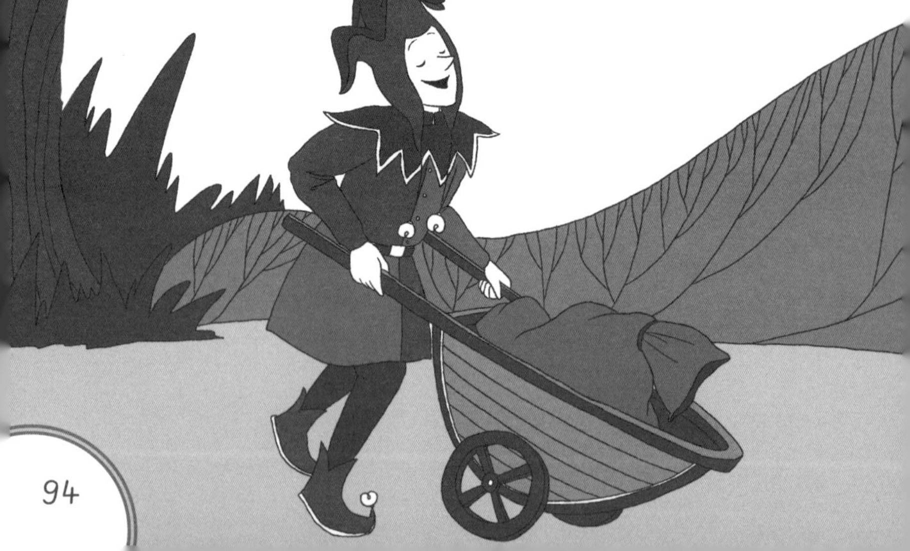

'Quiet! You are not helping,' said Kent, taking King Lear's arm to help him walk.

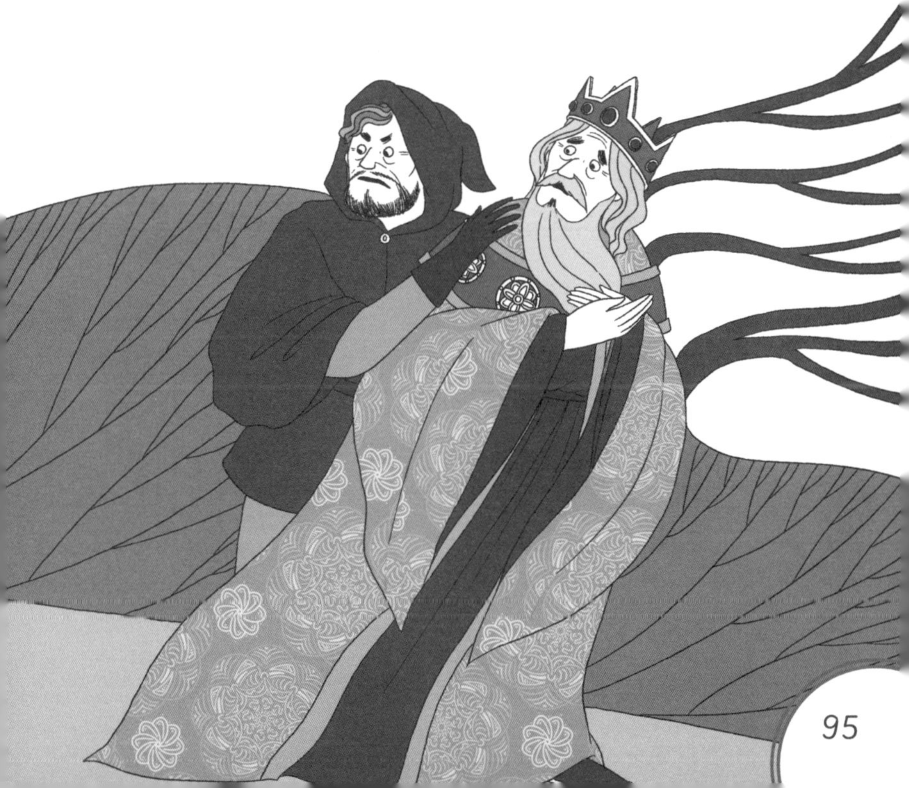

'He is right. I have been a foolish old man,' said King Lear sadly.

'It is not your fault, Your Majesty,' Kent said.

'My daughters were good,' said King Lear. 'I must have done something very bad for them to hate me now.'

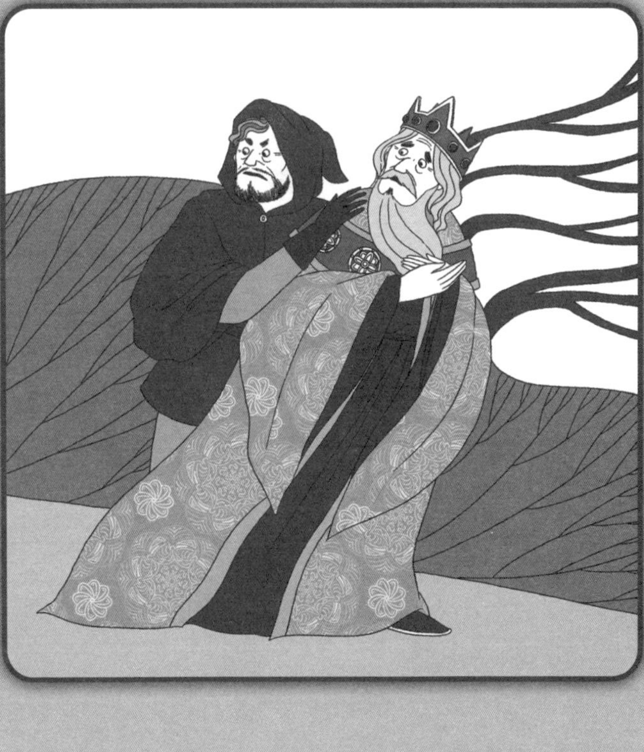

Kent knew it was time to tell King Lear who he really was.

'No, that is not true,' he said. 'Your daughters are **dishonest**. I knew it the day you gave your kingdom to them.'

King Lear was confused. 'But you weren't there,' he said.

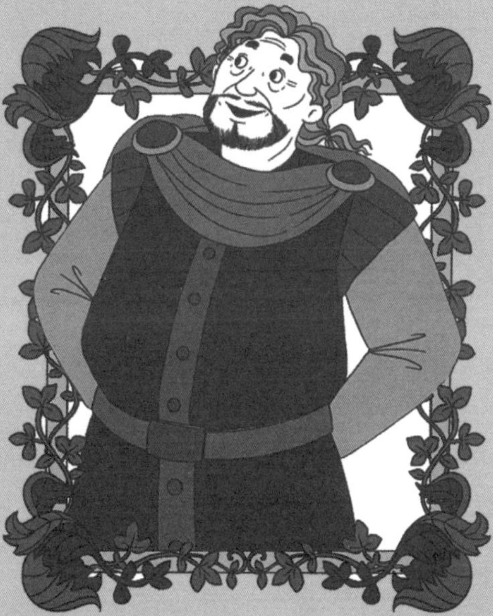

dishonest - Not telling the truth.

Kent took off his disguise. The jester laughed and began skipping around.

'Kent came back!' the jester said. 'Even though you told him not to!'

'Is it really you?' King Lear asked. 'But I treated you so badly!'

Kent nodded. 'I am your loyal friend, Your Majesty,' he said.

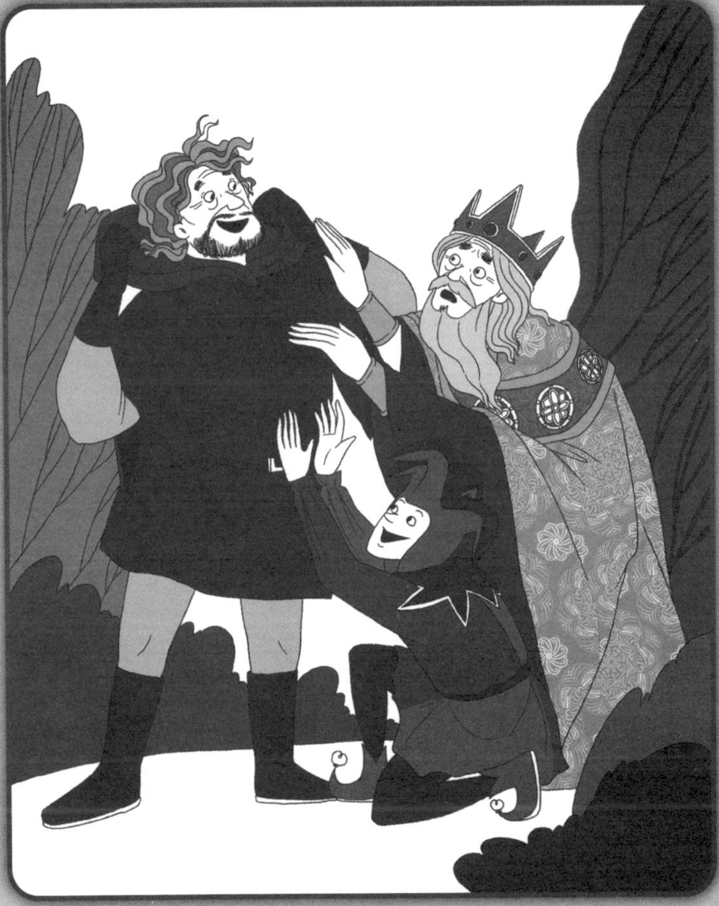

'Your daughter Cordelia and her husband are coming to help you,' Kent said. 'They will be here soon. They are ready to fight for you.'

King Lear's eyes filled with tears.

'You knew!' he said. 'Cordelia loved me the most! I have been so blind.'

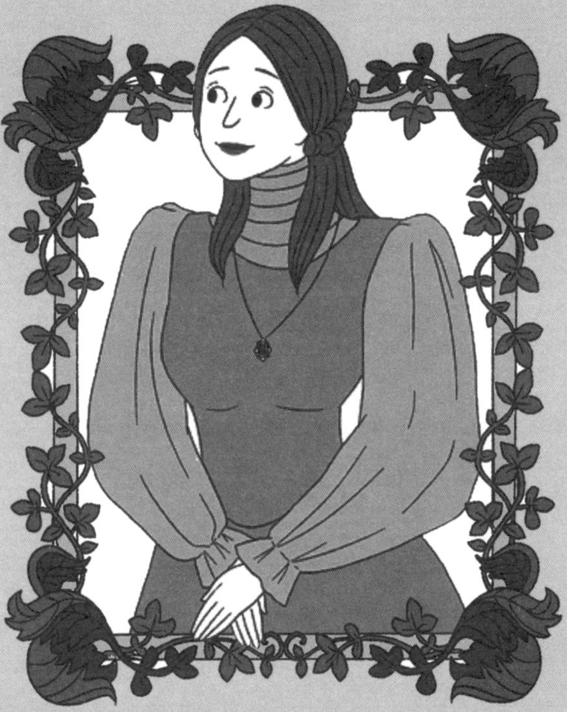

The sea off the coast of **Dover** was full of French ships.

Cordelia was looking out for her father, Kent and the jester.

'I have missed Father so much,' Cordelia said to the King of France.

Just then, she saw three people walking towards her. It was them.

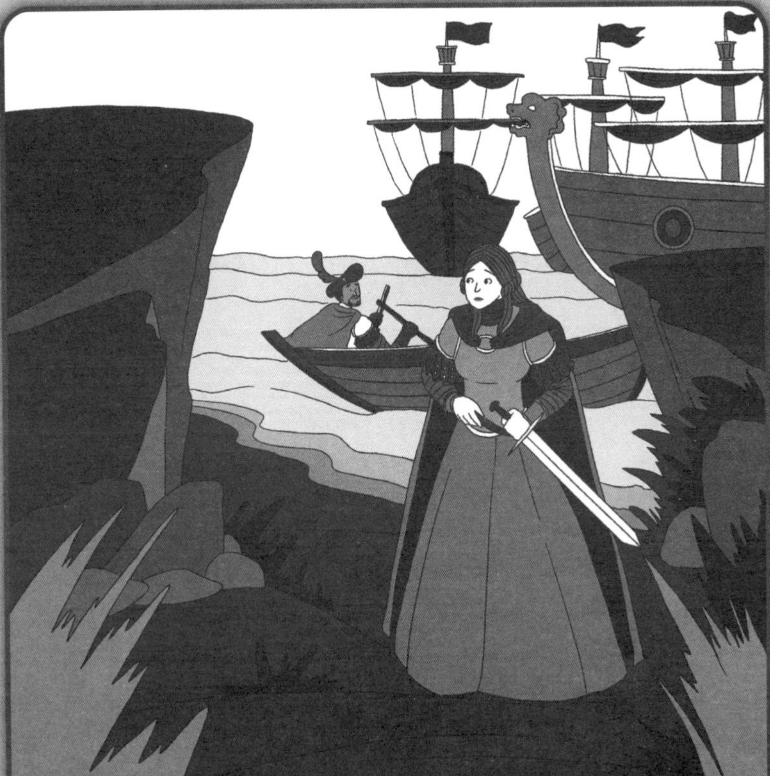

Dover - A town on the coast of the south of England.

Chapter 9

When Regan heard that Cordelia and the King of France had arrived, she sent for her sister, Goneril.

To win a battle against King Lear and Cordelia, Regan and Goneril needed to work together.

But the sisters argued.

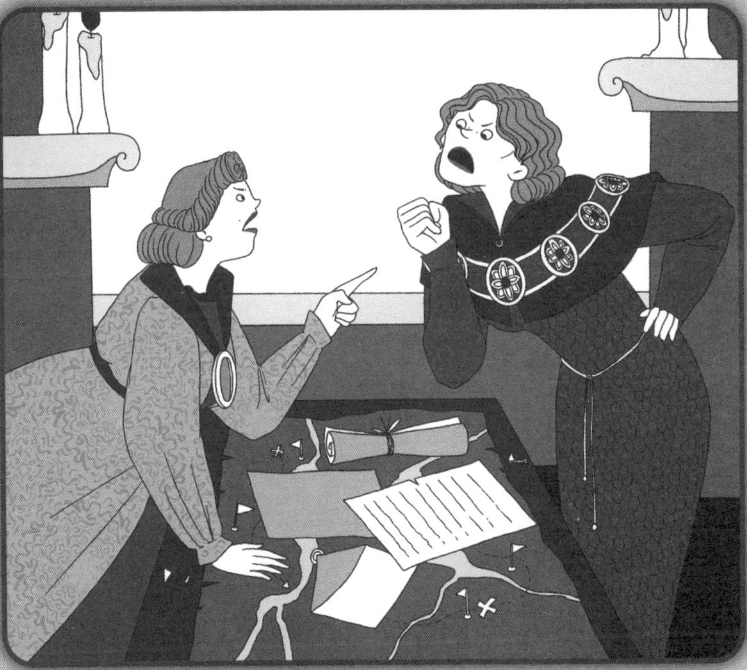

'I don't trust her!' said Goneril to her husband. 'Regan is going to try to take my half of the kingdom.'

'Isn't that what you are planning to do to her?' he asked.

Goneril smiled. She had got rid of her father. Now she would get rid of her sister.

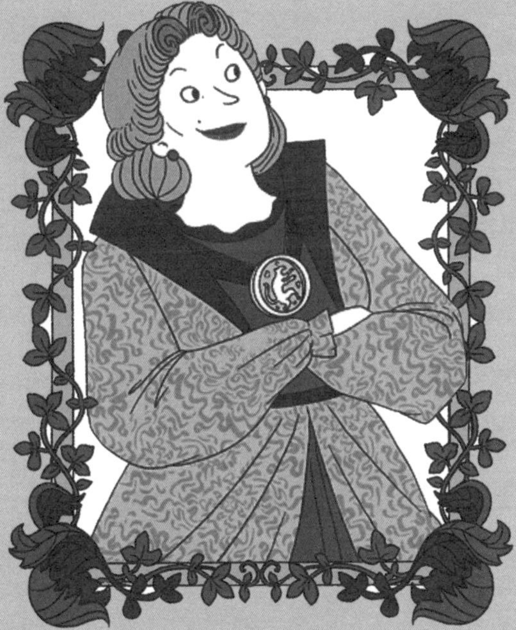

Goneril knocked on her sister's bedroom door.

Regan opened it.

'What do you want?' Regan asked.

'To say sorry,' Goneril replied, handing her sister a mug of warm milk. 'I brought you this to help you sleep.'

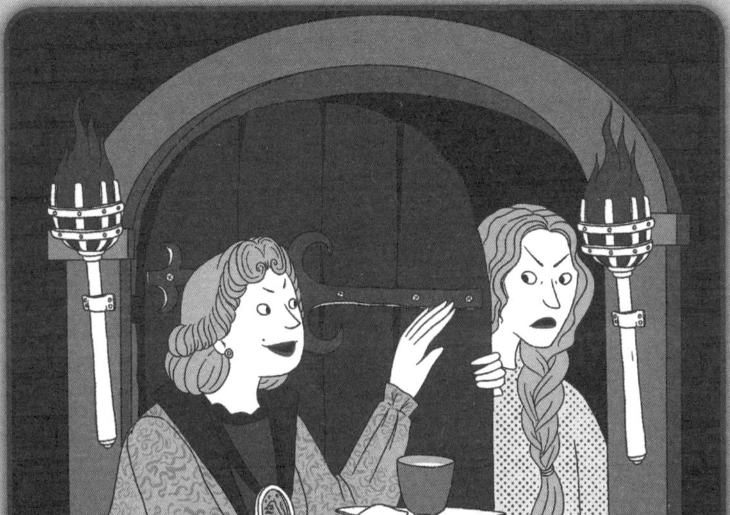

Regan took the mug from her sister.

'We must work together,' Regan said. 'Once Father and Cordelia are dealt with, the kingdom will be ours.'

Regan took a big sip of the milk. Goneril suddenly looked terrified.

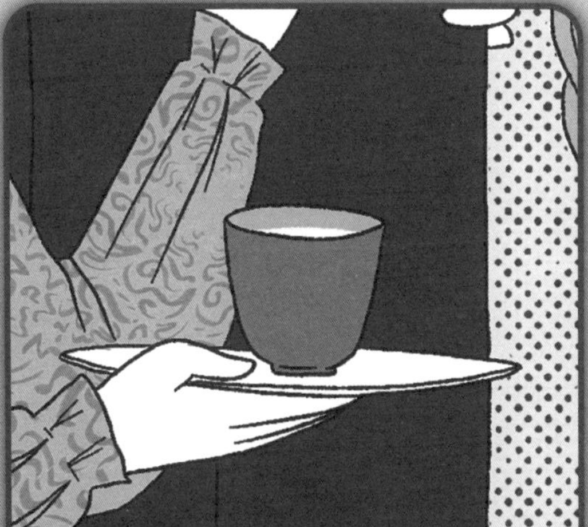

'Regan, wait!' Goneril shouted, **snatching** the mug from her sister's hands. 'Spit it out! I'm sorry! I should not have done it!'

But it was too late. Regan fell to the floor. She was dead, **poisoned** by her own sister.

'What have I done?' Goneril said, falling to her knees.

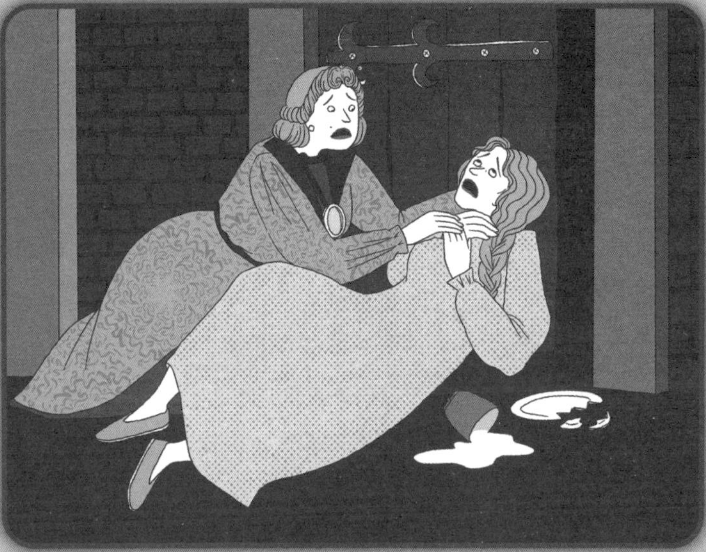

snatching - Taking hold of quickly and suddenly.

poisoned - When someone has been given something to eat or drink that has made them ill or killed them.

Chapter 10

Albany and Cornwall were on their horses. Behind them, their soldiers were ready to march into battle.

In front of them was the French army camp.

Somewhere in the camp were King Lear, Kent and Cordelia.

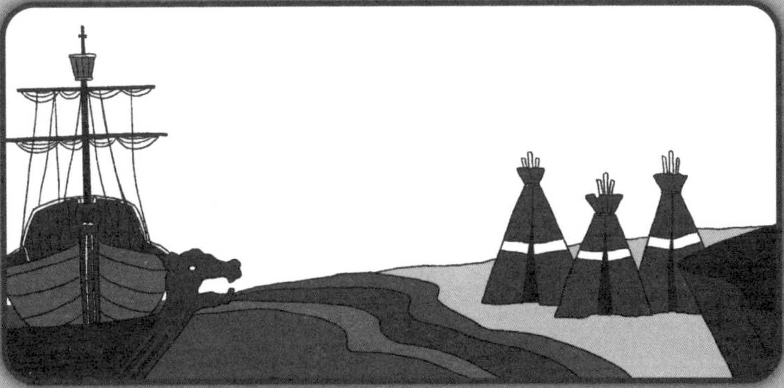

'I am sorry about your wife's death,' said Albany to Cornwall. 'But I am glad you are here.'

'My wife was **murdered** by Goneril,' Cornwall said. 'She wanted to make sure King Lear and Cordelia would not take her kingdom. I am here to do that for her.'

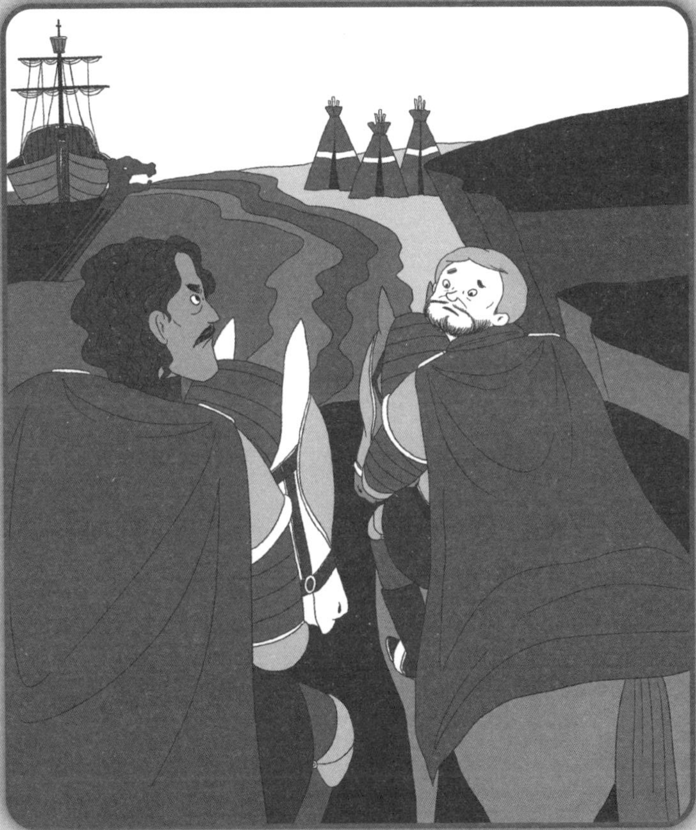

murdered - Killed on purpose.

Albany knew his wife had poisoned Regan. Goneril was behaving strangely. She did not sleep anymore. She just cried and talked to herself.

'My wife is very upset,' he said at last. 'Regan's death has made her dangerously ill.'

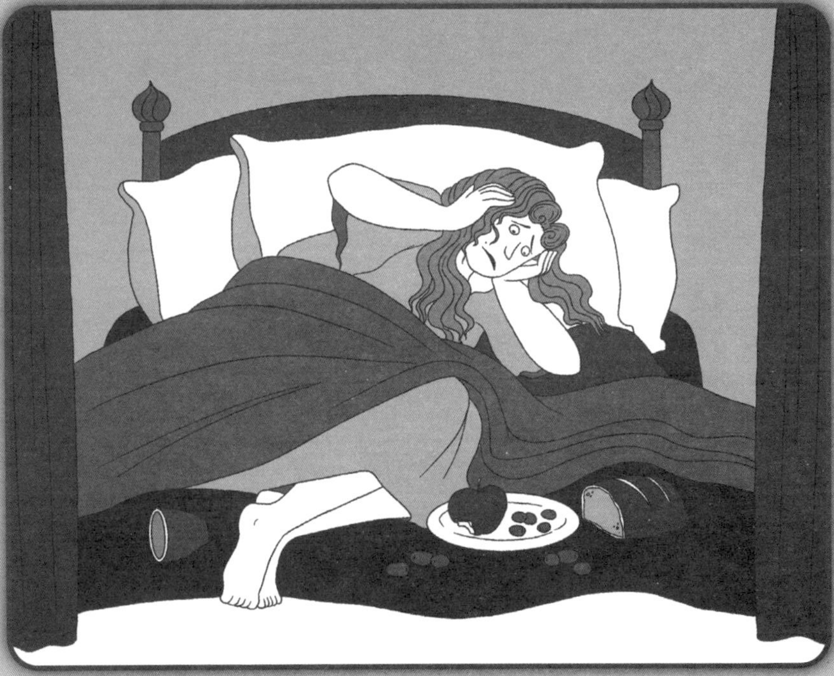

Cornwall stared at Albany. 'Good,' he said. 'It is no more than Goneril deserves.'

A flag was raised in the French camp, showing that they were ready to fight.

A huge roar was heard from the soldiers behind Albany and Cornwall. They charged forward.

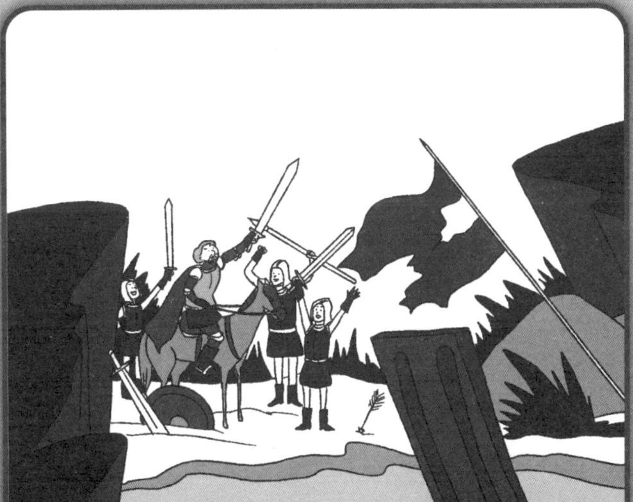

There was a huge battle.

The English soldiers fought hard. They were strong and skilled. They won the battle.

The King of France and the last of his soldiers escaped back to their boats.

The battle was over.

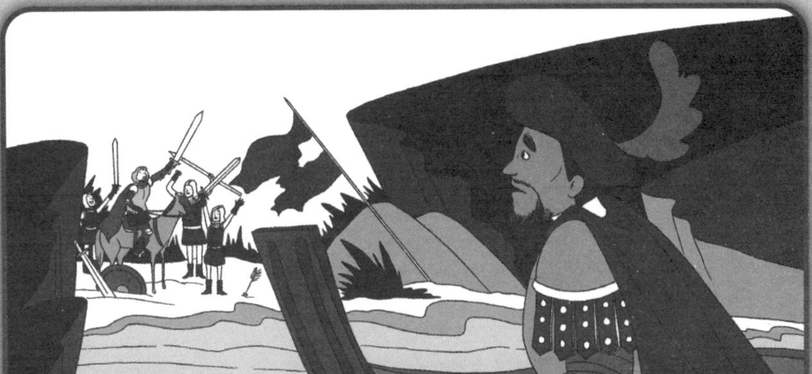

Albany had taken Cordelia and King Lear as his prisoners.

He should have been happy. But he kept thinking about Goneril. He wondered how she could have killed her own sister.

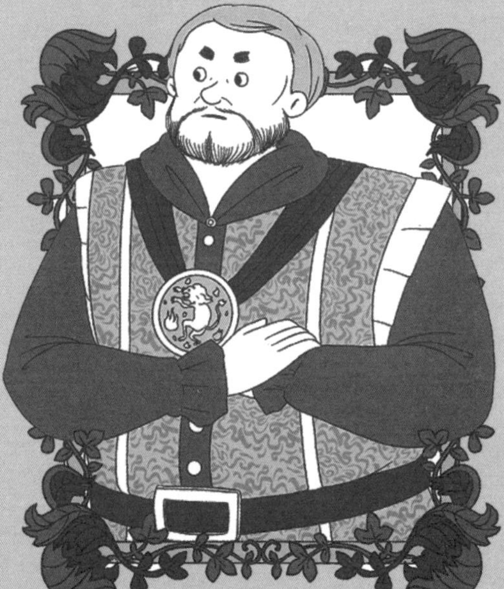

At that moment, a young soldier walked over to Albany. The soldier gave him a piece of paper.

'A message from your castle, sir,' the soldier said.

Albany read the message. Goneril had died.

Now that both his wife and Regan had died, who was left to rule over the kingdom?

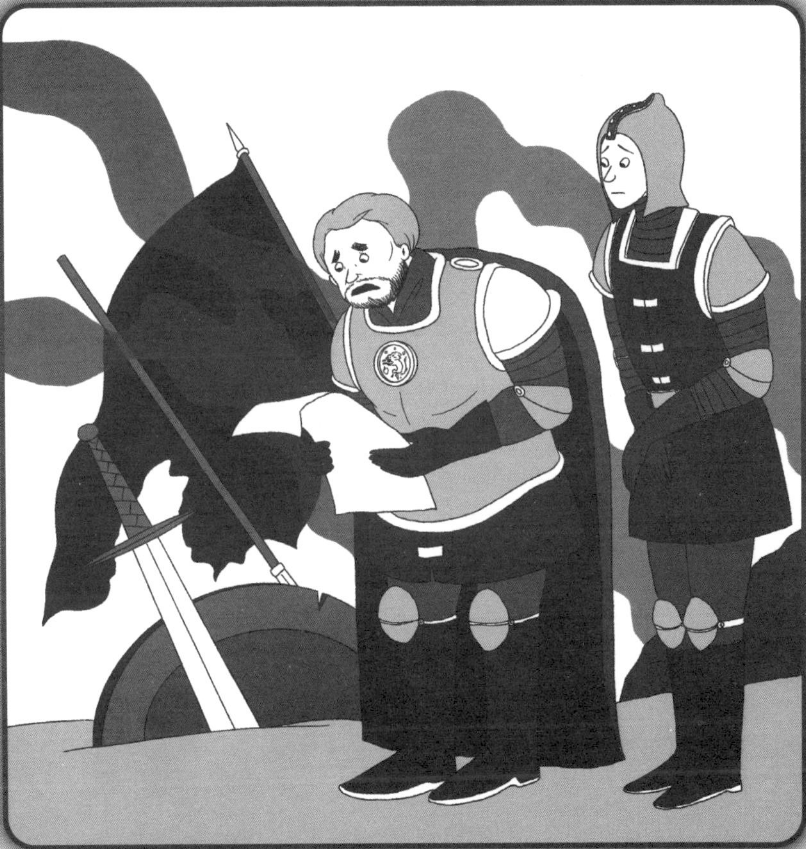

Cordelia would now be queen of the kingdom!

'You!' Albany said, calling back the soldier who had given him the message. 'Take me to Cordelia and King Lear. We have made a bad mistake!'

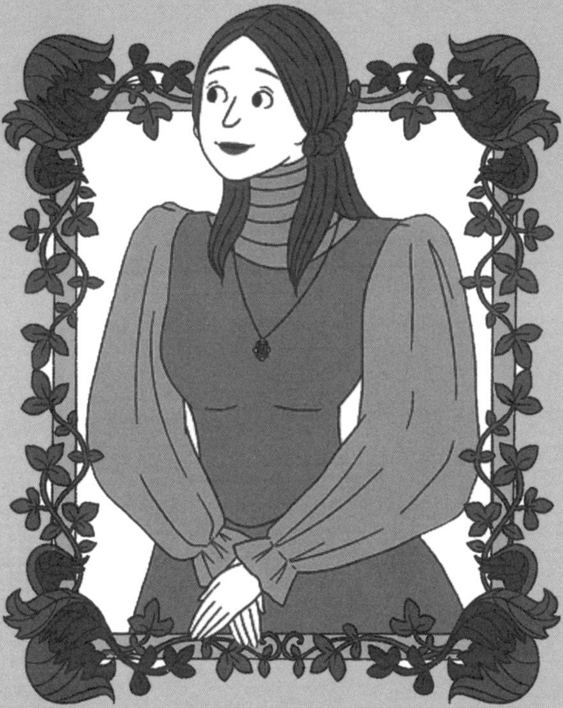

Chapter 11

Cornwall **stood guard** outside an old barn.

The barn was being used as a prison for Cordelia and King Lear before they could be taken to the castle prison.

Suddenly, Cornwall heard the loud noise of horses as Albany and the young soldier arrived.

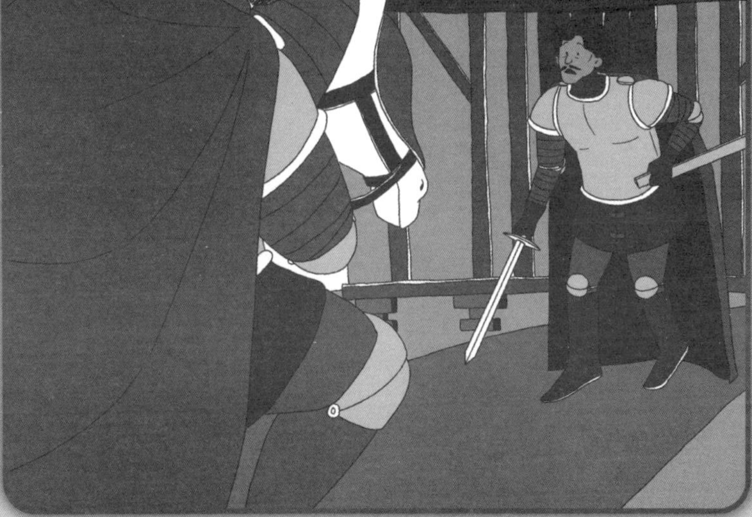

stood guard - Stood near someone to watch and protect them.

Suddenly - Quickly and not expected to happen.

'Goneril is dead,' Albany said, getting down from his horse.

Cornwall couldn't believe the news.

'But if Goneril and Regan are both dead, that means Cordelia is queen!'

The men rushed to open the barn doors to set their prisoners free.

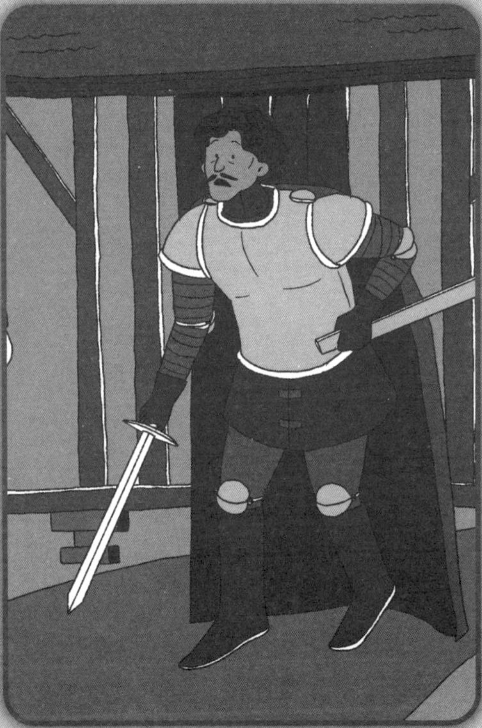

King Lear came out with Cordelia in his arms. Kent followed him and the jester came last. Both men stared at the ground.

'It is all my fault,' said King Lear, gently placing his daughter on the ground. 'If it wasn't for me, my daughters would all still be alive.'

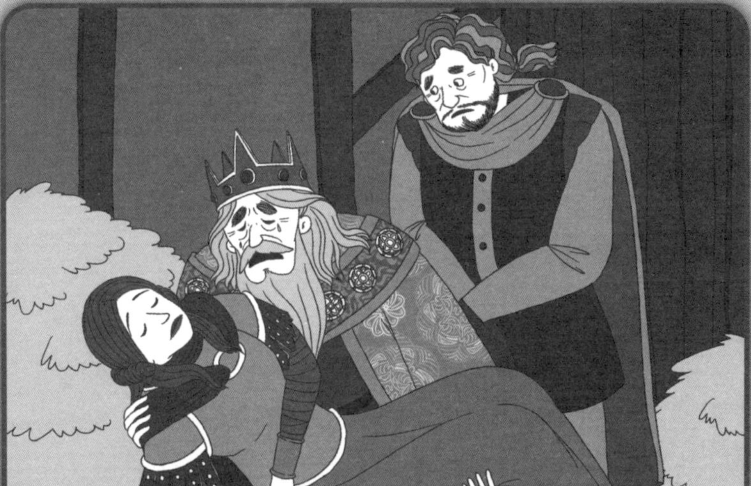

Cornwall and Albany looked at Cordelia. She had fought bravely in the battle but had been wounded. She had died in her father's arms.

'I know now that Cordelia loved me more than her sisters,' said King Lear, tears running down his face. 'I am such a fool.'

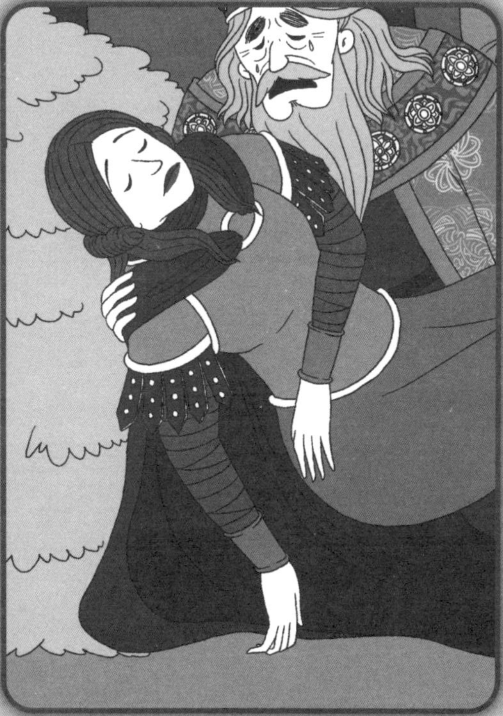

King Lear fell to the ground. His body shook as he cried for his daughter.

King Lear had no family and no kingdom.

He had nothing left to live for.

He died next to the daughter who had loved him the most all along.

The End.

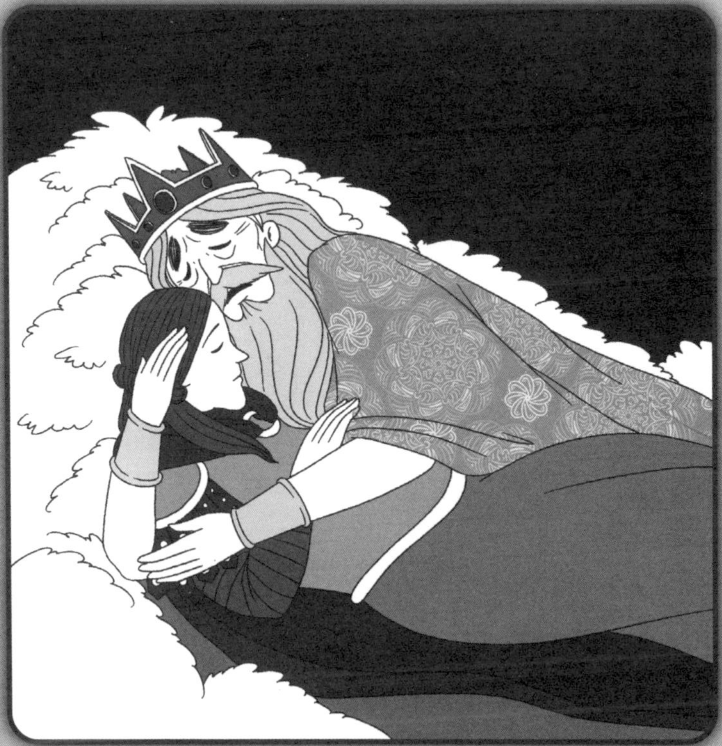

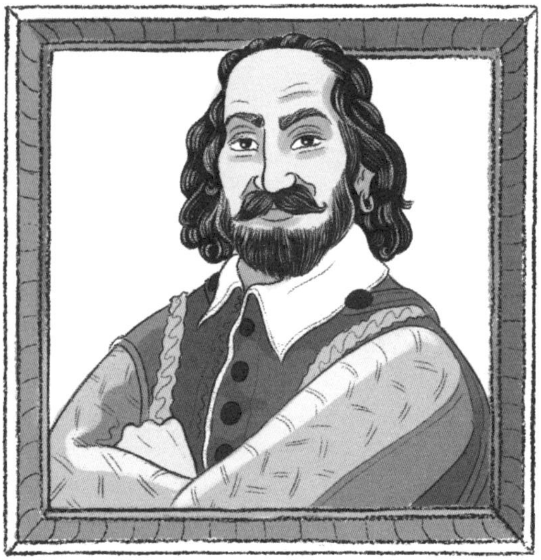

William Shakespeare

In 1564, William Shakespeare was born in Stratford-Upon-Avon, a small town in the West of England.

Shakespeare enjoyed writing plays and poems. He wrote 38 plays!

Queen Elizabeth the First loved to watch his plays. They were performed especially for her family and friends.